# PRAISE FOR TH

CW00696089

"A must read before you see your fertility ∶
ask all the right questions!"

**Dr Manuela Toledo**, *MBBS FRANZCOG MMed CREI, Fertility Specialist,
Gynaecologist, Melbourne IVF*

---

"This book has culminated decades of experience from a team
of incredible women and brilliant clinicians. I am thrilled to have read
this remarkably thorough book. I consider *Create A Fertile Life* the
new go-to resource for every couple on their baby making journey and
would recommend to both patients and health care providers alike".

**Angela Hywood ND**, *Naturopathic Clinician*

---

"This book will be an invaluable resource for couples looking
to conceive and have a healthy pregnancy."

**Dr Adam Watkins**, *Assistant Professor of Reproductive Biology, University
of Nottingham, Division of Child Health, Obstetrics and Gynaecology*

---

"I feel lucky to have been supported by the wonderful and
knowledgeable team at Fertile Ground Health Group for the past
12 months. A thorough preconception plan helped me to recently
conceive! I feel happy and confident that I am giving this little human
the best possible start to a healthy life. This book is the perfect
resource for anyone else on the same journey, that will not only
benefit your own health now but for generations to come."

**Kaitlin McMahon**, *Fertile Ground Health Group Patient, Holistic Nutritionist*

---

"For 20 years the extraordinary health professionals of Fertile Ground
have provided care as naturopaths and acupuncturists to my patients.
The evidence-based approach to their practice has provided me with
the reassurance that my patients, who almost always have high-risk
pregnancies, will receive safe, considered and compassionate care.
I commend this book to women planning or embarking on a pregnancy."

**Professor Mark P. Umstad**, *AM,MB BS, MD, FRCOG, FRANZCOG
Director of Maternity Services, Royal Women's Hospital, Melbourne*

"As a medical fertility specialist, many of my patients undergo treatment with other health professionals including naturopaths and acupuncturists. *Create a Fertile Life* has been written by the team from Fertile Ground to provide an invaluable resource for patients and clinicians alike. It is evidence based whenever practicable and I do not hesitate in recommending it."

**Dr David Wilkinson**, *MBBS BA FRANZCOG CREI PhD, Medical Director, City Fertility Centre, Melbourne*

---

"A truly holistic and comprehensive book on maximising fertility. I especially appreciated the scientific references and the advice on environmental health, sleep and nutrition".

**Dr Natasha Andreadis**, *MBBS MMed FRANZCOG CREI INHC, Fertility Specialist, Gynaecologist, Reproductive Endocrinologist and Clinical Lecturer at the University of Sydney, presenter of Dr Tash TV*

---

"A wonderful, thoroughly researched and easy to implement guide for anyone wanting to fall pregnant."

**Tasha Jennings**, *Author of* The Fertility Diet and Your Fertile Pantry

---

*Create A Fertile Life* is an excellent resource that combines scientific research with clinical experience and practical information to help you understand what you can do to boost your fertility and prepare your body for conception. I highly recommend it for anyone who is planning conception in the near future. The health and fertility questionnaires are a fabulous and fun way to really assess your health, personalise your experience and start to understand the factors that may be impacting your ability to conceive."

**Belinda Kirkpatrick**, *Naturopath, Nutritionist, Creator of Seed App for Fertility and Author of* Healthy Hormones - A practical guide to balancing your hormones

---

"With infertility on the rise, affecting even younger couples, it has become necessary to understand which factors are impacting fertility and the ability to carry a baby to term. In this day and age the information in this book is essential for anyone trying to conceive and wishing to create a healthy baby. There is no greater gift you could give your child than a robust health and to be able to do that you need to properly prepare for pregnancy."

**Iva Keene**, *MRMed. BHSc (Nat). ND, Natural Fertility Specialist and creator of Natural Fertility Prescription*

---

"The desire to have a child swells from our hearts and runs deep in our biology — perhaps it's our deepest drive. This comprehensive book, overflowing with expertise from naturopaths and acupuncturists who specialise in reproductive health, brings a depth of information to guide you towards your best health and wellbeing for conception, pregnancy and a healthy baby."

**Rhea Dempsey**, *Childbirth Educator, Birth Attendant, Counsellor and Author of* Birth with Confidence: Savvy choices for normal birth

---

"Here is the ultimate guide in understanding and working with your fertility. This book is the complete A to Z of fertility awareness with practical steps and ideas to help you achieve your goals. As a seasoned birth worker, this is my new go-to book for any couples wanting to conceive."

**Lael Stone**, *Founder and Creator of AboutBirth Online*

---

"A practical, reader-friendly, comprehensive guide to fertility - highly recommended for anyone trying to conceive."

**Dr. Leila Masson**, *M.D., MPH, FRACP, FACNEM, DTMH, Paediatrician & Lactation consultation and author of* Children's Health A to Z

---

*Create A Fertile Life* is a wonderful companion for any couple on their fertility journey."

**Lara Briden**, *Naturopathic Doctor, Author of* Period Repair Manual

---

"Read in as much detail as you need, be guided to find the information you seek and build a greater (broader) understanding of your fertility health. *Create A Fertile Life* is the collection of experience and information that women are seeking to empower their fertility journey."

**Dr Lionel Steinberg**, *Obstetrician and Gynaecologist*

---

Be Fertile Media · Melbourne

# Create a Fertile Life

**Everything you need to know to get pregnant naturally,** boost your fertility, prevent miscarriage and improve your success with IVF

Gina Fox, Charmaine Dennis
Rhiannon Hardingham
Tina Jenkins, Milly Dabrowski

Published in Australia by Be Fertile Media
Suite 603, 372-376 Albert Street, East Melbourne, Vic 3002

Email: *management@fertileground.com.au*
Website: *www.fertileground.com.au* and *www.befertile.com.au*

First published in Australia 2019
Copyright © Be Fertile Media 2019

For clinic, corporate or bulk orders contact our team by email at
*management@fertileground.com.au*

A catalogue record for this book is available from the National Library of Australia.

ISBN: 978-0-6483911-0-4 (paperback)
ISBN: 978-0-6483911-2-8 (Epub)

Cover design by Zahra Keramat
Book design and typesetting by Carla Thornton
Printed by IngramSpark

**Disclaimer**

This book is intended to provide helpful and informative material and is for
guidance only. It is not intended to provide medical advice and cannot replace
the advice of a health professional. The authors and publishers have, as far
as it is possible, taken care to ensure that the information is accurate and
up-to-date however new research is always emerging. No responsibility can
be accepted by the publisher or author for any damages resulting from the
misinterpretation of this work. The author and publisher shall not be responsible
for any person with regard to any loss, damage or injury caused directly
or indirectly by the information in this book.

be fertile
media

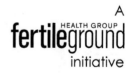

# DEDICATION

For the many thousands of courageous people we have seen who have attended in all the possible ways to their preconception health to benefit their health, fertility and baby-making potential over the past 18+ years. You have taught us so much about the struggles and challenges of infertility. This is for people just like you who are now starting at the beginning of this journey to improve their own outcomes and create their own healthy family.

# GRATITUDE

We are forever grateful to our mentors in this work who have taught us through their generous sharing of information and writing of books on the topic of women's health and fertility. Namely Francesca Naish, Ruth Tricky, and Jane Lyttleton. We also wouldn't be the practitioners we are without the support of Rachel Arthur and Kerry Bone.

Thanks to Foresight, the UK charitable organisation, who has been instrumental in championing and developing pre-conception health care over the past 30 plus years. Much of this information in this book originated from yes, their foresight, as well as passion for education on the many benefits of preconception health care.

We also want to thank those in the medical profession who are championing research in this area and spreading the word at fertility conferences too, namely Nick Macklon and Robert Norman along with the good people at the Australian government funded organisation Your Fertility (*www.yourfertility.org.au*). It is so good to see more and more evidence emerging and gaining traction among fertility specialists and IVF clinics every year in support of the things we have been saying for so many years.

# NOTES TO THE READER

We value inclusivity, diversity, and providing accessible information to everyone who wants to increase their fertility and start their healthy family. We want to be clear that this content is designed for everyone, no matter if you are a potential sole parent or in a relationship, the structure of your relationship or what orientation or identification you align with.

Over the years, alongside married, de-facto and living apart heterosexual couples, we have also supported single women, same sex couples, surrogates, women and men who are gifting donor eggs or sperm to other single women, non-binary people, single and partnered men, as well as now (and about time Australia) married same sex couples to conceive and bring beautiful babies into the world.

We have tried where ever possible to use inclusive language in this book, but as we can't acknowledge all of the possible permutations every time, we hope you can take the benefits of the information regardless of identification terminology used, and know we intend the best for you.

"DO SOMETHING
TODAY THAT YOUR
FUTURE SELF WILL
THANK YOU FOR"

SEAN PATRICK FLANERY

# CONTENTS

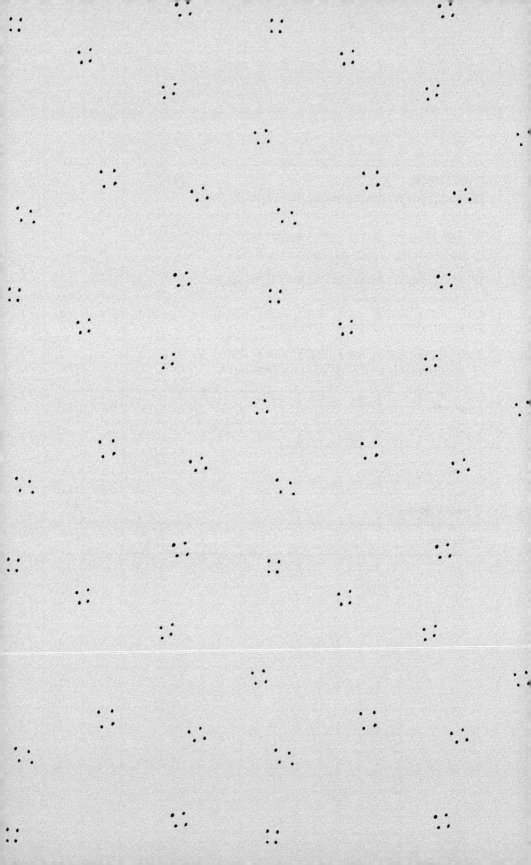

# About the authors

Charmaine Dennis founded our incredible collaborative health practice back in 2001 in a private maternity hospital in Melbourne. After the birth of her own healthy baby in 2003, she joined forces with Milly Dabrowski to form a highly creative partnership under the banner of one of their greatest accomplishments – Fertile Ground Health Group (FGHG).

Charmaine (a naturopath) and Milly (an acupuncturist) have over 45 years of experience between them working as health professionals, as well as individual experience across a broad range of areas from acupuncture, naturopathy, massage, and nutrition to journalism, meditation, marketing and public relations to personal development and business success, to yoga and birth attending. There is a rare depth and breadth of experience here that enriches every aspect of their work. In seeking a life of purpose and fulfilment, they followed their hearts with open curiosity to create a business beyond even their own expectations.

Charmaine continues practice and active leadership of FGHG and is committed to reaching out to form collaborative relationships with colleagues in Western medicine through public speaking, education and other relationship-building opportunities. She is also an enthusiastic mentor of practitioners and students to help them realise their full potential as natural medicine practitioners. Milly is now in private practice in country Victoria, following a tree change, her love for yoga and the eternal quest for a simpler life.

**Gina Fox, Rhiannon Hardingham, and Tina Jenkins** are all highly-qualified and experienced naturopaths with over 60 years of experience combined. They all have post-graduate qualifications in Natural Fertility Management. Gina and Tina also have a Masters in Reproductive Medicine from the University of New South Wales. They are all passionate writers, lecturers and mentors who walk their talk in their own lives and enjoy the many benefits of good health. As for all practitioners at FGHG, these three are highly collaborative and recognise the benefit of a supportive health-care team to suit an individual person's needs. Ideal outcomes are achieved for patients when all their health-care providers are working together. They work effectively alongside and in regular communication with many of Melbourne's most well-respected fertility specialists and obstetricians, expertly supporting couples and individuals with male and female infertility, IVF support, and pregnancy care. They all incorporate the use of herbal medicine, nutritional therapies and lifestyle counselling to achieve optimum results for each individual patient.

The team at FGHG have assisted many thousands of couples, same sex, and sole parents in achieving full-term pregnancies and beautiful healthy babies. Charmaine and Gina have also developed the Be Fertile series of guided relaxation CDs, created for women around conception, IVF, and pregnancy support. Rhiannon runs regular on-line naturopathic group mentoring and a masterclass in IVF support.

# WHO ARE FERTILE GROUND HEALTH GROUP?

As a leading natural medicine fertility clinic in Melbourne, Fertile Ground Health Group have some of the most experienced practitioners in the treatment of fertility, pregnancy, and family health. We are committed to providing expert care and compassionate support to help patients achieve their families.

Expert services include acupuncture and Chinese herbal medicine, naturopathic fertility treatment, IVF support, medical obstetric and gynecology services, pregnancy massage, osteopathy for mothers and babies, counselling and birth attendants/doulas.

Fertile Ground Health Group has the resources to meet the needs of men, women and couples wanting to get pregnant, those undergoing IVF, patients wanting to optimise their health in pregnancy, needing to prepare for labour or finding support for birth, the post-natal period or family health. Consultations are in our Melbourne office, or for patients further afield or in another country we have virtual online and/or phone consultations.

The ethos at FGHG is to have inspired, informed and passionate people working closely together, committed to motivating and educating ourselves, each other and our patients with the most current and well-researched approaches we can get our hands on. We want all our patients to receive the best care, and so work collaboratively both within our own clinic and with your other health-care providers. This makes for the safest and best treatment outcomes and it also makes this a truly great place to work.

*"I have been fortunate to work in a number of different clinics (both medical and complementary) in Australia and overseas. However, I can honestly say that I have never worked in such a collaborative team environment. FGHG is really unique in that it has brought together such an incredible level of highly-skilled, compassionate and experienced practitioners all with an amazing passion for fertility issues. In addition, all the support staff on reception and in management are the best I have ever worked with. It is no wonder that I often hear patients tell me of how happy they are to have found FGHG."*

**Tina Jenkins**, naturopath and author

# CONTRIBUTORS

Thanks to Josephine Cabrall for her great attention to detail, research insertion and fact checking. Josephine is a naturopath trained in natural fertility education and is the author of the *PCOS Solution*. She has a special interest in polycystic ovarian syndrome, fertility and pregnancy.

Thanks go to our colleagues at Fertile Ground Health Group (past and present) for their invaluable input. Sarah Harris, paediatric and family naturopath who contributed to the menu suggestions in the food chapters. Experienced fertility traditional Chinese herbalists and acupuncturists Rachel Steward gave advice on the Chinese medicine approach to fertility, and Amy Forth gave valuable input with recommendations and edits. Acupuncturist and Chinese medicine practitioner and presenter of Finding Fertility podcast, Joanne Sharkey, contributed to advice on research. Naturopaths Nicole Tracy and Samantha Van Dort contributed patient stories from their extensive experience as clinicians in this field. Gabrielle Covino, naturopath and clinical supervisor, gave editing support and review of the food chapters, and naturopath, nutritionist and lecturer Ljupka

Peev added research and editing to part 1. Thanks for the expert contribution of Nicole Bijlsma, a building biologist, author of *Healthy Home, Healthy Family* and a researcher in the field of how chemicals impact our health. Nicole gave advice and edited our chapter on the Environment.

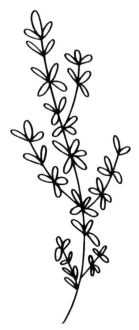

"THE KEY TO REALISING
A DREAM IS TO FOCUS NOT
ON SUCCESS BUT SIGNIFICANCE
– AND THEN EVEN THE SMALL
STEPS AND LITTLE VICTORIES
ALONG YOUR PATH WILL TAKE
ON GREATER MEANING"

OPRAH WINFREY

# Let us inspire you

## HOW TO CREATE
## A MORE FERTILE LIFE

### Kylie's Story

*Kylie came to see us after 9 months of trying to conceive. She complained of weight gain (her BMI indicated she was 10-12 kilos overweight), sugar cravings and recent blood tests indicated she was pre-diabetic. In addition, Kylie also had food intolerances to dairy and wheat. Due to her regular consumption of these foods, she experienced multiple digestive symptoms including constipation, indigestion, and heart burn. Her energy was low, and she struggled to get out of bed in the mornings.*

Kylie experienced long menstrual cycles (36 days) with cervical fertile mucus apparent around Day 19 as well as PMS symptoms including tearfulness and irritability.

Kylie's job was quite stressful and involved long hours, which frequently resulted in her reaching for unhealthy foods, leading to her weight gain. Although she was overwhelmed with her health and felt down about her weight she was determined to fall pregnant, which motivated her to change her diet and lifestyle.

Her naturopath designed a diet high in protein, vegetables, and good fats with some additional whole grains to help shift Kylie's excess kilos and improve her energy levels and fertility. She also removed dairy and wheat to ensure her digestion was functioning properly, resulting in an almost immediate improvement in her digestive symptoms. Kylie was advised to always carry healthy snacks (with a list of ideas provided to her) and looked at healthy meal options when she was very busy at work. As Kylie needed extra support to help balance her blood-sugar levels, herbs and supplements were prescribed that helped reduce her sugar cravings and supported her nervous system during times of stress. Kylie also began a regular exercise routine and enlisted the help of a personal trainer to help achieve her weight-loss goals.

Within a month Kylie had mastered her diet and was finding she had far less sugar cravings than before. Within six weeks she felt she could avoid processed sugar almost completely. Kylie had also started to lose weight and felt she had more energy every day. By the two-month mark, Kylie's menstrual cycle had reduced in length to her first ever 29 day cycle and this was maintained for the following three months, indicating an improved hormonal balance. During this time Kylie had also lost seven kilos. She fell pregnant the following month and went on to have a healthy baby boy.

CREATE A FERTILE LIFE

The irony is that having a baby seems as simple as falling off a log – in fact, it seems so easy most people spend the majority of their adult lifetime trying to avoid falling pregnant! It is a bitter pill indeed when it turns out that fulfilling that dream doesn't happen so easily.

If you are reading this book, you probably already know the facts around the increasing rates of infertility in the general population, which is around one in six couples experiencing fertility issues: 35% due to women's reproductive issues, 21% due to male factors, 12% combined male and female, and 28% of infertility cases have unknown causes.[1-3] Infertility is a challenge for couples (as well as single people or same sex couples trying to conceive), regardless of who has the diagnosed issue, and especially if the fertility problem is unclear.

There is no doubt that trying to conceive is an incredibly emotional and stressful journey for couples to whom it does not come easily. Family-making seems like a birth right and it feels unjust when this right appears to be denied. And the worst thing is that if you are having trouble conceiving, it appears that absolutely everyone around you is pregnant – older women, young women, women who weren't trying, women finally achieving their miracle baby ... it can be unbearably frustrating, even devastating for some to celebrate another's joy when they are facing a future without children.

Many couples end up feeling isolated, alone in their grief, trauma, struggle and stress and ultimately, helpless. Seeking the one magical answer that will provide the solution becomes an obsession for some women (and men) as they spend hours online with others in similar circumstances looking for answers.

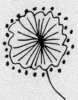

# ALL CRISIS HAS THE POTENTIAL TO TRANSFORM

One of our favourite sayings is: "all crisis leads to transformation".
You may see this as another useless platitude, or it could be a mantra
that leverages you out of helplessness and into a shift of perspective
to identify what this opportunity means to you, and how to make the
most of it. This struggle can leave you unchanged, or it could be your
greatest teacher, giving insight into what makes you feel good, what
a truly healthy lifestyle is, what is damaging your health, well-being
and fertility and, most importantly, how to make lasting change that
will affect not just your health, but that of your whole family – possibly
for generations to come!

Our work focuses on the care of those struggling with fertility issues:
people who long to make a family. In providing health solutions to
fertility problems and improved overall health to enhance fertility,
we have supported many women and men in their journey to create
a healthy family. While we like to think of our work as preventative –
the ultimate pre-conception care is being as healthy as possible before
even starting to try to conceive – most often we are working with
individuals and couples with complex diagnoses or unexplained fertility
issues. In most cases, we identify and support practical changes that
can be made in health and lifestyle to dramatically improve the health
of a couple and optimise their chance of conceiving.

When they first start trying, many people think they are 'healthy
enough' to conceive, but sadly in some cases good enough is not
enough to get across the line. Each person is unique and responds
to all that life throws at them differently. While one couple seems to
have a poor lifestyle and are able to conceive, another feels they are
much healthier yet still struggle. It doesn't seem to make sense and
it certainly doesn't seem fair.

# HOW YOU CAN IMPROVE YOUR FERTILITY EVEN WHEN DOCTORS SAY YOU CAN'T

If you have undergone IVF treatments, you will know just how important creating a quality embryo is to achieving a pregnancy. If you are trying to conceive naturally, this still stands. It is estimated that over 90% of genetically normal embryos will result in a live birth, whereas at least half of all miscarriages are due to chromosomally abnormal embryos.[4] Therefore, achieving that quality embryo is the first step in every successful parenting journey.

But what is the 'perfect embryo'? Does it mean you'll have good looking, smart children who have inherited all your best bits, and none of the 'bad'? Not at all. Both the egg and the sperm contain 23 individual chromosomes, which combine at the moment of conception to create the 23 pairs of chromosomes required to make a human. At the very moment conception occurs, your child's genetic stamp – the strongest predictor of their future health, learning abilities and susceptibilities – is created. These outcomes are dictated by those individual 23 chromosomes in the sperm and the egg.

When this is understood, the reasons for preconception care are more obvious. Both the sperm and egg take around three months to develop/mature, and in this time they are both vulnerable to damage, creating interruptions to normal, healthy development and even chromosomal abnormalities. The embryo and developing baby are significantly influenced by their environment and their genetic development is profoundly altered by outside influences. So we focus on reducing risk factors, optimising the environment in which they develop and hopefully creating the most positive outcome possible: a sweet, healthy baby.

> Preconception planning directs us away from unquestioning or despairing acceptance of genetic destiny or environmental randomness. Investing in yourself during this time of your life goes a very long way. There is surely no other time in which such major changes occur and where our action is potentially most powerful.

Our lifestyles, diet, toxic load and life stages play a significant role in influencing the expression of our genetic code as new cells are made. It seems it is not such a lottery after all. Healthy choices can strongly impact your chances of conceiving a healthy baby – and even your baby's chances of healthy fertility! There are many well-known and medically-researched factors that impact directly on your fertility and outcomes, such as smoking, drinking alcohol, being overweight or underweight, advancing age, certain environmental and home chemical endocrine disruptor exposure and other factors you will read a lot about in this book. There are also many factors that, while not directly affecting your fertility, can have an indirect effect. Things like chronic health problems and complaints (digestive problems, periodontal health, asthma, sleep issues, stress, nutritional factors, even emotional considerations) may add up to an unhealthy load that compromises the whole organism and puts fertility right at the bottom of your bodily priorities – even in so called healthy individuals. Certainly, starting your pregnancy from a basis of optimal health will help to ensure minimal pregnancy discomforts and disease as well as positively impacting on the health of your developing baby at every crucial stage.

Preconception health really does set the foundation for creating healthy eggs and sperm to conceive and have a healthy pregnancy and baby. So what does it involve? Ideally for at least three to four months before you begin trying to conceive, you will both pay close attention to your diet and lifestyle, your environment, and chronic health issues that need to be addressed. Extensive testing for nutrient levels, gland and organ function, infections, heavy metals and other contributing factors are all undertaken. Your family history is explored, and your personal medical and health history is extensively mined for clues as to anything that may compromise your fertility. Everything from impotence to nutrient deficiency, hormone imbalance to urinary tract infections can all be important contributors to fertility, many of which are highly treatable or responsive to natural medicine support. This process is comprehensive, enlightening, empowering and most importantly takes you on a journey of continuous improvement that at the very least leaves you feeling healthy, energised and vital, and may help you achieve a healthy baby.

## IS THIS INFORMATION REALLY IMPORTANT FOR MEN TOO? (ISN'T FERTILITY A "WOMEN'S PROBLEM"?)

The truth is, male fertility is declining at such a rapid rate that it is not just an issue for up to 50% of couples experiencing infertility, it has become a real public health issue. Sperm concentrations in Western men have declined 50% over the past 40 years according to a recent research review.[5] Particularly associated with advancing age, lifestyle, diet choices, and environmental factors, the consequences on the future of human population is concerning to say the least. The information we share here is so important for men to embrace - environmental, nutritional, physical exercise and psychological support, combined with the use of appropriate supplementation. Attention and focus here can really improve semen parameters and prevent infertility, improving the chance for a couple to conceive spontaneously or optimise their chances of conception.[6-8]

> Where possible, attending to preconception health for at least three months prior to sperm collection is just as important for men donating sperm too.

In our experience, men are not always on board with exploring this territory let alone committing to all the changes. They may be too confronted or embarrassed or just unwilling to wade through this kind of information about health and fertility like women often are. We also know that some men see how their sperm is a reflection of their overall health and they are really ready to make change and prevent more potentially serious health consequences in the future – as well as improve their sperm health, fertility and health outcomes for their baby too. When men get on board with this, we do see time and time again how important it is for the women they are making babies with. When men make a concerted effort to help improve their own fertility and the healthy conception and pregnancy outcomes, women feel so supported, so much more able to adhere to the recommendations themselves, and as an added bonus, of course it is good for the relationship too!

To make it easy, read the questionnaire section first to find out the most important information required, and then look at the Top Tips section at the end of every chapter. That way you can get straight to it. If it doesn't make immediate sense to make the changes suggested there, go back through the chapters for more information and plenty of science to back it all up too.

# WHY READ THIS BOOK?

In this book we're going to discuss what YOU can do to increase your chances of success. At first it may seem overwhelming to incorporate these changes into your life but by breaking down the process into clear steps and applying the practical tips outlined in this book, you may be pleasantly surprised by your own capabilities. Importantly, the benefits will speak for themselves.

We aim to give guidance to maximise your health and well-being so that fertility can regain its place nearer the top of your physical hierarchy. We focus on the key factors that improve your chances of conceiving a healthy baby. We shed light on the changes you can both immediately and gradually incorporate into your life that will impact positively on your fertility. We focus on what you can do and give you direction when you might need a little extra help. Of course, age is an issue we will discuss, but there is not much any of us can do about the fact that we are getting older. However, what you can do is stop the things we know (or will find out here) that make us age more quickly and in a more unhealthy way. We can put aging on a little holiday by embarking on a super regime of health that maximises the vitality and function of every cell in your body – right down to the microscopic little eggs and sperm that will one day be your baby!

## AN ADDED BONUS

Your fertility is a barometer of your general health. As well as an increased chance of conceiving a healthy baby, this approach promises a host of other benefits. All treatment approaches have their side effects and ours is no different. Reported effects have included: improved aging (anti-aging), increased energy, healing or improvement of chronic health issues, stress reduction, weight loss, sleep enhancement, reduced disease risk, especially for some of the most common lifestyle diseases including diabetes, cardiovascular disease... and so much more! The investment you make in your health now will have consequences well into advanced age.

Health costs are not going down so investing in health now is cheap compared to what it will cost you to manage poor health in 10, 20, 30 years' time. And of course, your healthy baby is less likely to bring a swathe of health-related bills and time off work for you in its wake.

The most current research in the area of genetics shows that your choices now can have an influence for generations to come. This is a further amazing opportunity. Being in the position to choose consciously, to take up this opportunity to be your healthiest, wisest, most knowledgeable, fit, energised, healthy-weight self before you get pregnant means you get to create the legacy of health for yourself and your partner, your children and even of generations to come.

Creating a fertile life might be just the ticket to not only getting what you ultimately want, but creating a lasting outcome that remains a gift to your family for generations.

## IF WE DO THE WORK, WILL I GET PREGNANT AND HAVE A HEALTHY BABY?

We are often asked by patients what the odds are of their falling pregnant, what our success rate is. These are fair questions but not straight-forward ones to answer. Unlike a running race, the fertility journey for most people is not a straight run to the finish line. But very much like a running race, those who do well are usually the ones who have put in the hard yards: done the training, eaten well, taken care of themselves, made adjustments along the way, done as their team of experts has advised and consequently showed good endurance.

Sadly, we know not everyone who comes to our clinic is able to do this work. There are numerous reasons: either it doesn't resonate with them, they don't 'believe' in it (even the scientific research cannot convince them), they don't want to make changes such as giving up alcohol, coffee, or changing their diet and lifestyle; they don't have time, or they've already tried so many things...

What we do find is that those who allow us to come on the journey with them — providing support, advice, encouragement and guidance on making changes and who really implement the recommendations and take their supplements and yucky tasting herbs — are the people who most often find success. We are happy to say that most of our patients who make the necessary changes do have positive outcomes.

# Claudia's Story

*Claudia was 39 years old, with a 5-year-old son and was desperate to add to her family. She booked a consultation after having two miscarriages, which were followed by two unsuccessful IVF stimulation cycles. Claudia had had an incredibly rough couple of years. She was feeling a pregnancy was never going to happen, and her AMH (Anti-Mullerian Hormone is one way to measure a woman's ovarian reserve) level was less than one, indicating a very low number of remaining eggs.*

*Claudia was keen to undertake naturopathic pre-conception care, making the dietary and lifestyle changes outlined in our book. She also took the supplements and herbal tonic we prescribed for the next three months in the lead up to her final round of IVF. Claudia was very diligent with taking the prescribed medicines, and felt a huge lift in her energy levels and libido, and a significant drop in stress levels and anxiety. Her husband also made changes to his diet and took prescribed nutrients during this time.*

*Nearing the sixth week of treatment, Claudia voiced her concerns about re-embarking on IVF treatment. She was very reluctant to put herself through more failed attempts, but endeavoured to put her fears aside as her desire to grow her family was so strong.*

*Three weeks later, Claudia called to advise she was pregnant. This happened naturally, before her IVF was scheduled. On her first scan, it was discovered that she was having twins!*

The most important thing we know is: 'There is nothing good health is not good for.' Nothing. The healthier you are mind and body, the more likely you are to be successful in any endeavour. This does not mean if you have a health condition of some kind that you won't be successful. It is simply about optimising, creating the best you, making the most of what you've got. And amazingly, it is not that hard. You'll feel better, happier, more resilient – no matter what disappointments or challenges might come your way.

## WHAT ARE YOU WAITING FOR?

Your fertility challenges can be the turning point of your life. A point you look back on and say: "that is where I chose to make it all different." A year from now, you will wish you had started today!

You may have picked up this book hoping to find out what pill to take or what therapy to undertake that will help you to conceive tomorrow. Sadly, that just isn't possible – there really is no such thing as a magic bullet. You may not be aware that you are in the midst of one of your biggest opportunities ever! Amazing opportunity often comes cleverly disguised as a major, painful challenge, which can make it hard to see where the opportunity bit comes into it. If you are reading this book, chances are one of these opportunities is presenting itself to you! Finally, you have the chance to really shine and be your best – and what better inspiration than the creation of your potential baby?

As you may have gathered by now, this book is all about you and what you can do to create a fertile life. We will be here to help you along this path – whether you're our patient or just reading our book. At the end of each and every day, this is your opportunity, these are your outcomes to create.

# How to use this book

This book provides the building blocks to understand where you sit currently with your general and reproductive health, then motivates and informs your choices to live a healthier, more fertile life. Start by completing the health and fertility self-assessments to direct you to the chapters that will be most relevant for you. Of course, you can always work your way through the book from front to back, but we have tried to provide some guidance as to the most important sections for you and your individual circumstances so you can jump right in to what is most important for you. As practitioners, we are always trying to assess what factors are most likely to be impacting your fertility and begin working through the most important first. This is what we want you to do too.

**Part One** of the book is a fertility masterclass, which will give you practical information and suggestions you can immediately implement regarding your lifestyle, exercise, sleep, stress and environment. Part 1 is relevant to everyone.

**Part Two** of the book is also a must-read for everyone, inspiring a fertility-boosting diet and recommendations for healthy digestion and eating.

**Part Three** is most relevant for those who may have more specific health conditions related to reproduction such as pre-menstrual syndrome (PMS), polycystic ovarian syndrome (PCOS), endometriosis or thyroid issues; and for people in their mid to late thirties or older, as fertility is compromised by age. It is also recommended for those with less than optimal general health, for example: allergies, fatigue, food cravings, inflammation, and digestion or weight issues. In many cases, there is no need to feel defeated by your circumstances, as there is plenty you can do to help get the best outcomes.

You will find a 'Top Tips' section at the end of each chapter to give you a summary of the most important points so if you haven't read the chapter in detail you can get started on these immediately. These tips are also a good reference for you to revisit a month or two into your journey to ensure you are maintaining the necessary changes.

## IS THERE ANY RESEARCH TO SUPPORT WHAT WE DO?

There is an overwhelming body of evidence to support our recommendations and we have tried to include as much research as we can. By no means is this exhaustive, nor is this book intended to be a scientific literature review. Between our busy practices, we have been writing this for over 6 years now, back and forth between us all. Much of it comes from what we have learned from medical and complementary medicine studies, as well as our combined experience supporting people trying to conceive every day in practice. There may well be research that we didn't see and even more research that comes out after the day we stop writing. We have done our best to include as much relevant research as possible.

We know it is so helpful for some people to see that there is evidence to back up what we are saying. We know others find the suggestions to be common sense and worthy of making change regardless of the evidence. We have tried to appeal to both.

What is true, is that each piece of evidence shows some improvement in outcomes, and when you add them all together, each of those gains can really add up to make the difference you need to create your healthy baby. Personal and professional experience tells us that it can feel overwhelming, isolating and lonely trying to navigate all of this on your own. Experience also tells us you'll cope better and have better health outcomes when well supported by a professional team who know the terrain. Hopefully the work we offer helps to cut through some of the darkness.

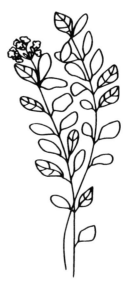

# Health and fertility self-assessments

## ASSESSING YOUR OWN FERTILE POTENTIAL

Start with these fertility health self-assessments and then jump straight into the chapter where you need the most focus. Be honest with yourself when answering the questions. We recommend you repeat the assessment after reading the chapter and implementing some change. That way you can be motivated by your steps in the right direction, give yourself a pat on the back where you see improvements, and know if other strategies are needed to take you to the next level of health.

# Self-assessment 1:
## Sex and timing

Essential information to ensure you are trying to conceive at the right time of your cycle.

| DO YOU: | YES | NO |
|---|---|---|
| Have sex at least three times a week on average? | | |
| Rely on an App to tell you when you ovulate? If so, then give yourself a 'No' | | |
| Try to conceive in the two days before ovulation or on the day of ovulation? | | |
| Know when you ovulate or when your fertile window is? | | |
| Know what fertile mucus feels like and notice it during your cycle? | | |
| Use a sperm-friendly lubricant? If so, then give yourself a 'No' | | |
| Know statistically what your chances of conception are each month? | | |
| Have a regular menstrual cycle between 26-33 days? | | |
| Know that you may not ovulate on Day 14? | | |
| Understand how to chart your menstrual cycle with mucus and temperature changes and know how to interpret the information? | | |

**SCORE:** 8-10 'Yes'

It sounds like you do know how your hormonal cycles work, although in an Australian study it was found that lack of fertility awareness was a cause of infertility with only 13% of the women in the study accurately pin-pointing their fertile window even though 70% thought they knew.[9] Did you know that studies show many apps are incorrect and only average your cycle giving you your incorrect ovulation date? As our vaginal pH is so important to safeguard the sperm, it may mean that even sperm-friendly lubricants are best left out. So you might just want to glance through the Sex and Timing chapter to check you are correct.

**SCORE:** 2 or more 'No'

As getting the timing right is one of the key factors to successful conception, then Sex and Timing is definitely the chapter to begin reading immediately. If you can learn more about your menstrual cycle and ovulation, it's been shown that pregnancy rates increase significantly.

# Self-assessment 2:
## Smokes, booze, and caffeine

When you are trying to conceive these are the things that are, in most cases (apart from medical necessity), non-negotiable. To get an idea of your actual consumption of these we recommend you keep this diary for a week and discover how you rate.

| SUBSTANCE | NUMBER OF TIMES IN A WEEK | OPTIMAL FERTILITY CONSUMPTION |
|---|---|---|
| Alcohol (standard drink) | | Zero |
| Smoking | | Zero |
| Marijuana | | Zero |
| Other party drugs | | Zero |
| Over the counter drugs | | Only when medically necessary. Ask your GP and pharmacist for extra assurance of safety when trying to conceive. |
| Prescribed medication | | Take as prescribed by your doctor, ensuring they understand you are trying to conceive, and double-check with your pharmacist that it is safe for you and your baby. |
| Coffee | | Women: zero<br>Men: one per day maximum |
| Decaffeinated coffee | | Women: zero<br>Men: one per day if water-filtered decaffeinated. |

**SCORE:** 0 on all categories

That's fantastic! If you have been free of these substances for three months or more, you are all set to try to conceive without the hindrance of any negative effects of drugs, alcohol, and caffeine. No need to read the chapter on Smokes, booze, and caffeine unless you feel you need extra information and motivation to keep you on track.

**SCORE:** If you haven't scored 0 (or maximum seven (one a day) for coffee for the man) then we suggest you turn to read our Smokes, booze, and caffeine chapter to understand why we make these recommendations and get some tips on cutting down and quitting the substances that are likely adversely affecting your fertility.

# Self-assessment 3:
## Am I at a fertile weight?

Are you over or underweight? Or, in a good healthy range? Here are two useful markers for you to help work out if focus is required here - Body Mass Index (BMI) and Waist To Hip Ratio (WHR).

## 1. WORK OUT YOUR BODY MASS INDEX (BMI)

For the fastest results, use Google™ to find an easy BMI calculator and plug in your measurements. For the math geniuses among you though...

| WEIGHT (KILOGRAMS): | HEIGHT (CENTIMETRES): | TOTAL BMI |
|---|---|---|
|  |  |  |

**Your Body Mass Index = Weight/height$^2$**

(weight in kilograms and height squared in metres)

e.g. Weight 76kg, Height 162cm (=1.62m) 76/1.62 x 1.62 = 76/2.62 = 29 BMI
This example fits the overweight category.

The total BMI number number gives you a rough guide but doesn't suit all body types so please use common sense. Generally, for fertility for both men and women, you don't want to fall in the underweight or overweight / obese categories.

> ### BMI RANGES
> **< 18.5**: underweight | **18.5 – 25**: normal weight
> **25 – 30**: overweight | **30-35**: obese | **> 35** morbidly obese

# 2. WAIST TO HIP RATIO (WHR)

Another useful tool to gauge your health is a hip to waist measurement. This can be a better guide for some people. How much body fat you have around your waist can directly impact your fertility and indicate an increase in a number of health risks (including high blood pressure, Type 2 diabetes and heart disease).

**Waist measurement:**
While standing, relax your stomach and measure your waist at the halfway mark between the bottom of the ribs on the side of the body and the top of the hips.

---

**HEALTHY WAIST MEASUREMENTS:** [10]
**Women:** under 80 cm   |   **Men:** under 94 cm

---

**Hip measurement:**
While standing, measure your hips at the widest part.

**WHR = waist cm/hip cm**
Now, to get the waist to hip ratio number, divide your waist circumference by your hip measurement.
e.g. If your waist was 83cm and your hips 93cm then your WHR = 0.89

---

**WAIST TO HIP RATIO TO AIM FOR:**
**Women** less than 0.8   |   **Men** less than 0.9

---

| WAIST (CENTIMETRES): | HIP (CENTIMETRES): | WHR |
|---|---|---|
|  |  |  |

A waist/hip ratio (WHR) of under 0.8 (and ideally 0.7) for women and 0.9 for men has been shown to correlate with general health and fertility. Women with a WHR higher than 0.8 have lower pregnancy rates, and men with WHR higher than 0.9 have been shown to be less fertile.[11-13]

# WHAT DOES THIS MEAN FOR ME?

**BMI under 18.5**

Look at ways to increase your weight through a healthy diet (read up on Food in Part 2), consider your exercise, sleep and stress (Part 1) to help pinpoint any other factors that may be impacting your weight.

**BMI between 18.5 and 25 and WHR less than 0.8 (women) or 0.9 (men)**

Looks like your weight might be just right for your body type. It appears weight isn't impacting your fertility, but it will still benefit to read the chapter and feel clear about what kind of exercise will keep you on track to support your health and fertility for the longer term.

**BMI over 25 and/or WHR over 0.8 (women) or 0.9 (men)**

Please read the chapter on Exercising for Fertility (Part 1) and turn to the Food section (Part 2) for ongoing healthy eating. If you tend to have a craving for carbohydrate or sweet foods or suffer with an inflammatory condition, our chapters about blood-sugar, inflammation and balancing your hormones (Part 3) will also be informative.

If your BMI or WHR is outside normal range, consider seeing a counsellor and naturopath or nutritionist to give you a helping hand, and to see if there are any other health issues affecting your weight. If you are overweight, a personal trainer or other motivational exercise specialist may also be considered for part of your health-care team.

# Self-assessment 4:
## Exercise – too much, too little or just right?

## HOW IMPORTANT IS EXERCISE TO YOU?

☐ Extremely important

☐ Very important

☐ Moderately important

☐ Slightly important

☐ Not at all important

As a basic rule for your fertility, if you rate exercise as extremely important you probably need to do less. If it's not important or only slightly then our guess is that you need to do more!

First keep this exercise diary for one or two weeks and then make an intention for future exercise levels. Your future plan should take into account whether you are looking to manage your weight, feel more energised, or improve mood. Also make a note if you feel more energised or exhausted after exercise. If you feel exhausted afterwards, you may need to pull back a little and improve other areas of your health before increasing your exercise.

Record any physical movement into your diary including dance classes, yoga, exercise classes, swimming, sport, weights, walking the dog, tennis, golf, physical work in the garden, gym etc. Even make note if you walk up and down the stairs at work. How many levels can you walk before stopping? Does it improve over time?

# ACTIVITY DIARY – TYPICAL WEEK

| DAY | ACTIVITY | HOW MUCH TIME SPENT (MINUTES) | INTENSITY* |
|---|---|---|---|
| Monday | | | |
| Tuesday | | | |
| Wednesday | | | |
| Thursday | | | |
| Friday | | | |
| Saturday | | | |
| Sunday | | | |

* Intensity: Low is walking when breathing is easy; moderate is a step up like brisk walking, swimming, dancing, golf, social tennis, pushing a pram or medium weights; high intensity is where you will be breathless and working up a sweat such as aerobics or interval training, jogging or running, fast cycling, carrying a load or digging.

# AM I EXERCISING ENOUGH?

Current health guidelines suggest that we should be active on most days of the week.[14] Are you doing the minimum scheduled exercise of 2.5 to 5 hours per week of moderate intensity activity? Or 1.25-2.5 hours of more vigorous high intensity activity? Or a combination? It is also recommended you do muscle strengthening activity two days a week. Break up prolonged sitting by working at a standing desk or building in times to get up and move during the day. For example, your ideal may be a combination of 45 minutes of low intensity (walking) on most days of the week plus two to three sessions of higher intensity or muscle strengthening exercise.

If you are reaching these targets and you don't need to manage your weight, then well done and keep it up or mix it up to make it more enjoyable. If you're falling short, then now's the time to strengthen your resolve and turn to the chapter on exercise to get some inspiration. Read the chapter (in Part 1 on exercise and fertile weight) and complete your "intention to exercise" (see below). Follow this up with noting how your week might look with your intended exercise routine and make it achievable. You might build this up each week. Complete the Activity Diary again after you have made these changes to ensure you are achieving the exercise you need to enhance your fertility.

My intention is to exercise _____ days a week and I will include the following in my exercise routine:

- o   i.e. one hour pilates class x 2
- o   i.e. walking the dog for 30 minutes x 3

- o   _____
- o   _____

- o   _____
- o   _____
- o   _____
- o   _____

# Self-assessment 5:
## Stress and emotional health

How are you coping at this point in your life? This assessment can give an indication of how likely it is that stress is impacting on your health, which may have a negative impact on your fertility.

| | YES | NO |
|---|---|---|
| Have you experienced any of the known major stressors in the past year:<br>o   Marriage?<br>o   Moved or renovated home?<br>o   Injury, illness or a medical diagnosis?<br>o   Infertility diagnosis or ART/IVF?<br>o   Job loss?<br>o   Death or illness of a friend or family member?<br>o   Divorce or separation? | | |
| Do you often feel nervous, low in mood or depressed? | | |
| Do you often wake in the middle of the night or too early in the morning? | | |
| If you wake before rising time, do you have trouble getting back to sleep? | | |
| Are you easily irritated, short-tempered or feel cranky? | | |
| Do you work long hours or in a high-pressure job? | | |
| Do you often reach for stimulants such as coffee, alcohol, drugs, tobacco? | | |
| Do you often feel overwhelmed? | | |
| Do you have a busy mind and tendency to worry? | | |

| | YES | NO |
|---|---|---|
| Do you feel there aren't enough hours in the day? | | |
| Do you have little energy for anything outside of work? | | |
| You don't do fun things anymore and have lost the joy in life? | | |
| Do you have no time to prepare and eat healthy food? | | |
| Have you experienced changes in appetite (especially not feeling hungry), regularly skip meals, overeat, or are you an emotional eater? | | |
| Are you on a mobile or other device at all hours of the day and night? Do you use your device to fill in the spare moments? | | |
| Do you have no time for exercise? | | |
| Do you often feel tired and emotionally exhausted? | | |

We know that stress impacts on our health and has a negative effect on our fertility. Research has confirmed a link between high stress and poor conception outcomes, both when trying to conceive naturally and with IVF. If you have been trying to conceive for longer than you were expecting, it can be hard to know if stress is a cause of your fertility issues or your fertility issues are causing your stress. Of course, telling you to relax does not help!

If you have answered yes to any of these questions, or if you do feel anxious, sad or depressed we suggest you head straight to our befriending stress chapter (Part 1). It may just give you a new take on enjoyment in life. If answering any of these questions has raised any concerns, please seek support or, in Australia call Lifeline on 13 11 14, or Beyondblue on 1300 224 636.

# Self-assessment 6:
## Sleep – am I getting enough?

Think about how you have slept for the past month and then complete this questionnaire.

| DO YOU: | YES | NO |
|---|---|---|
| Usually take longer than 15 minutes to get to sleep? | | |
| Often wake in the middle of the night? Have difficulty returning to sleep if woken before rising time? | | |
| Often wake to go to the bathroom? | | |
| Often wake early in the morning (this does not include being woken by an alarm clock)? | | |
| Generally sleep less than seven hours? | | |
| Snore loudly, have difficulty breathing at night or experience restless legs at night? | | |
| Often use a phone, computer, tablet or TV in bed? | | |
| Experience pain at night? | | |
| Feel too hot or too cold during the night? | | |
| Often experience bad dreams? | | |
| Often need to take sleep medication (prescribed, herbal or over the counter)? | | |
| Often wake unrefreshed? | | |

| DO YOU: | YES | NO |
|---|---|---|
| Often feel tired the following day and have difficulty staying awake? | | |
| Have a usual bedtime after 11.30pm? | | |
| Rate your general sleep quality as poor? | | |
| Frequently feel tired after a poor night's sleep? | | |
| Regularly need to nap in the afternoon? | | |

Sleep has a major impact on all aspects of our health with more than a few consequences for fertility too. It should be thought of as a daily vitamin we can't do without.

If you have answered yes to any of these questions, then it is likely your sleep needs your attention! Have a look at our chapters on sleep and stress (Part 1), and do seek help if you feel you need it.

# Self-assessment 7:
## Environmental and household toxins

How much potentially harmful environmental toxins are you exposed to?

| DO YOU: | YES | NO |
| --- | --- | --- |
| Eat organic food less than 70% of the time? | | |
| Eat tinned/canned food more than once a week? | | |
| Eat tuna, swordfish, shark, orange roughy or barramundi more than once a month? | | |
| Drink unfiltered tap water regularly? | | |
| Drink bottled water or use a plastic water bottle? | | |
| Have soft drinks in aluminium cans more than once a month? | | |
| Drink decaffeinated coffee? | | |
| Use non-stick cookware pans? | | |
| Store, heat or freeze foods in plastic containers? | | |
| Use cosmetics daily – face creams, make-up etc? | | |
| Use tinted lipstick? | | |
| Use an antiperspirant? | | |
| Dye your hair? | | |
| Use teeth-whitening products? | | |

| DO YOU: | YES | NO |
|---|---|---|
| Use perfume? | | |
| Have furniture less than two years old? | | |
| Renovate? Have you renovated in the last two years? | | |
| Smoke or are exposed to passive smoking? | | |
| Use cleaning products that contain fragrances? | | |
| Use laundry powder and dishwasher powder/liquid that contain fragrances? | | |
| Dry clean your clothes? | | |
| Use air fresheners? | | |
| Carry your mobile phone in your pocket? | | |
| Charge your mobile phone on your bedside table? | | |
| Have any appliances within two metres of your bed (think mobile phone, cordless phone, digital clock radio, wireless router, any bluetooth or wireless devices, remote controls, television, laptops, tablets and consider what is behind the wall in the next room too)? | | |
| Use an electric blanket? | | |
| Have a fuse box or house smart meter or meter panel close to your bedroom (check on the outside of the house)? | | |
| Fly regularly? Interstate or overseas? | | |
| Get exposed to toxic paints, glues, dyes etc or other chemical substances in your work? | | |

| DO YOU: | YES | NO |
|---|---|---|
| Get exposed to herbicides or pesticides when you garden or at work? | | |
| Live within one kilometre of a farm that uses pesticides? | | |
| Live within 200 metres of heavy traffic? | | |
| Live within 600 metres of high voltage power lines or five metres from street power lines? | | |

**SCORE:** Yes to 3 or less

If you ticked 'no' to the majority of these then you're on track for a healthy home and work environment. We still recommend that you check out this chapter on building a safe environment for your fertility as you might find there are some things in your environment you weren't aware could adversely impact your fertility.

**SCORE:** Yes to 4 or more

If you ticked 'yes' to four or more of these then start by reading the chapter on building a safe environment for your fertility (Chapter 7), and make a list of things you want to change. No need to be hard on yourself if you ticked lots of boxes — now is a great time to start making changes. Even if those changes are small, it's about getting on the right track — each change adds up.

# Self-assessment 8:
## Optimal nutrition for your fertility

Does your diet suit your body, and does it cover all the key food groups needed to enhance your health and fertility?

Complete this over the next week and see how you rate.

| FOOD | YES | NO |
|---|---|---|
| Do you eat at least 3 cups of varied vegetables most days? | | |
| Do you eat 2-3 pieces of fruit most days? | | |
| Do you eat whole grains (e.g. brown rice, wholegrain bread, rolled oats etc) at least once a day and not more than 3 times a day? | | |
| Do you have fish 2-4 times a week? | | |
| Do you eat chicken or white meat 2-4 times a week? | | |
| Do you eat red meat 2-4 times a week or less? | | |
| Do you eat eggs 2-7 times a week? | | |
| Do you eat dairy foods (e.g. cow's milk, yoghurt, cheese) 2-7 times a week? | | |
| Do you eat pulses such as lentils and chickpeas at least twice a week? | | |
| Do you eat a small handful of raw, unsalted nuts or seeds most days? | | |

| FOOD | YES | NO |
|------|-----|-----|
| Do you use olive oil, coconut oil, macadamia oil or butter for dressings, cooking etc? | | |
| Do you treat yourself to cakes, biscuits, lollies, or chocolate less than twice a week? | | |
| Do you drink soft drinks or fruit juices less than once a fortnight? | | |
| Do you eat refined white bread/rice/pasta once a week or less? | | |
| Do you add sugar to drinks? | | |
| Do you eat deep-fried foods less than once a month? | | |
| Do you order take-away food once a month or less? | | |
| Do you drink between 1.5-3 litres of water daily? | | |

**SCORE:** All yes

If you ticked all 'yes' then keep up the good work and continue to focus on the quality of your food instead such as choosing mostly organic.

**SCORE:** 2-5 'no'

Turn to Your Fertility Diet section (Part 2) first to give you more detail about our recommendations.

**SCORE:** 6 or more 'no'

It's time to take action and make changes to your diet as a priority. Turn to Your Fertility Diet section (Part 2) for more detail on improving the quality of your food and how and why we suggest you eat or avoid certain foods.

If you're a vegetarian/vegan or if you have food sensitivities, then you may be avoiding certain food groups and will need to make up for this with other food choices. We also suggest you read the Your Fertility Diet chapter.

If you feel you are sensitive or allergic to certain foods in particular, or worry that your diet may be causing some of your symptoms, check out the section on fast and challenge diets in the Inflammation chapter (Part 3) for a great tool to understand your food sensitivities.

# Self-assessment 9:
## Gut health and the microbiome

How we digest our food is one of the keys to our nutritional status and impacts our health significantly on many levels, including our fertility.

| | YES | NO |
|---|---|---|
| Do you get abdominal bloating after meals at least once a week? | | |
| Do you get indigestion or abdominal cramps at least once a week? | | |
| Do you experience fullness for an extended time after meals? | | |
| Do you experience gurgling in your stomach after eating? | | |
| Do you experience burping often? | | |
| Do you have a bowel motion less than once a day? | | |
| Do you have more than three bowel motions each day? | | |
| Is the consistency of your bowel motion loose (watery or like toothpaste) or hard to pass? | | |
| Do you ever see blood in your stool? | | |
| Do you ever see undigested food (apart from corn) in your stool? | | |
| Do you experience excessive or odorous gas? | | |
| Do you suffer from acid reflux/heartburn regularly? | | |
| Do you often feel nauseated after eating fatty foods? | | |

| | YES | NO |
|---|---|---|
| Do you have known food allergies? | | |
| Do you often feel fatigued after eating? | | |
| Do you have stomach upsets easily? | | |
| Do you have a poor appetite? | | |
| Have you taken antibiotics in the last year and not taken probiotics for at least six weeks afterwards? | | |

**SCORE:** 0 'Yes'

If you answered 'no' to all the questions, then your digestion is functioning well and you can skip reading the section on digestion. However, if you use medication for reflux or other bowel issues, this is a good section for you to prioritise.

**SCORE:** 1 or more 'Yes'

The more 'yes' boxes you ticked, the more you need to focus on your digestion. While it is ideal to answer 'no' to all questions, even one or two of these issues may mean your digestion is impacting your overall health and fertility. We recommend you turn to the chapter, Gut health, the microbiome and your fertility (Part 2), and begin to make the recommended changes. As a result, you may then enjoy improved digestion resulting in more stable energy and other health and fertility benefits. Once you've implemented some of the suggestions, try this self-assessment again in another month and see what improvements you've experienced.

# Self-assessment 10:
## Health issues that are impacting your fertility the most: hormones, blood-sugar, inflammation and ageing.

Part 3 of this book is based on particular conditions or symptoms and balancing your hormones. If you answer yes to any of these questions, then highlight or circle the ticks associated with the question and calculate your score at the end.

| | HORMONAL IMBALANCE | BLOOD-SUGAR | INFLAMMATION | AGING |
|---|---|---|---|---|
| Have you recently come off the oral contraceptive pill or other hormonal-based contraception? | ✓ | | | |
| Would you say your life and moods are ruled by your hormones? | ✓ | ✓ | | |
| Do you have an irregular or absent menstrual cycle? | ✓ | ✓ | | ✓ |
| Do you suffer most months from pre-menstrual symptoms such as moodiness, depression, breast tenderness, bloating, sugar craving, headaches, acne etc? | ✓ | ✓ | ✓ | |
| Do you experience spotting before your period or experience heavy bleeding or clotting at your period? | ✓ | | ✓ | |

| | HORMONAL IMBALANCE | BLOOD-SUGAR | INFLAMMATION | AGING |
|---|---|---|---|---|
| Do you have a menstrual cycle under 26 days or over 31 days? | ✓ | ✓ | | ✓ |
| Do you have an absence of fertile mucus during your cycle? | ✓ | | | ✓ |
| Do you know if you have 11 days or less after ovulation before you get your period? | ✓ | | | |
| Have you been diagnosed with endometriosis, fibroids, cystic breasts? | ✓ | | ✓ | |
| Have you been diagnosed or suspect you have polycystic ovarian syndrome (PCOS)? | ✓ | ✓ | ✓ | |
| Do you have excessive hairiness, particularly on the chin, upper lip, abdomen, and around the nipple? | ✓ | ✓ | ✓ | |
| Do you find it difficult to put weight on or to lose weight? | ✓ | ✓ | ✓ | ✓ |
| Do you often get painful periods? | ✓ | ✓ | ✓ | |
| Do you carry weight around your abdomen and hips? Or are you overweight? | ✓ | ✓ | ✓ | ✓ |

| | HORMONAL IMBALANCE | BLOOD-SUGAR | INFLAMMATION | AGING |
|---|:---:|:---:|:---:|:---:|
| Do you have low sexual desire, vaginal dryness, or night sweats? | ✓ | | | ✓ |
| Have you been diagnosed with a thyroid condition or sub-optimal functioning thyroid? | ✓ | | ✓ | |
| Do you have a consistent waking temperature of less than 36.3 or more than 36.8 between your period and ovulation? | ✓ | | ✓ | |
| Do you have increased sweating, night sweats or heat intolerance? | ✓ | | ✓ | ✓ |
| Do you feel the cold easily? | ✓ | | ✓ | |
| Do you suffer from generalised fatigue? | ✓ | ✓ | ✓ | ✓ |
| Do you often have cravings for sweet foods or carbohydrates? | ✓ | ✓ | ✓ | |
| Do you ever experience shakiness or feel faint if you haven't eaten for a while or are you hypoglycaemic, insulin resistant or diabetic? | | ✓ | ✓ | |
| Do you eat lots of carbohydrates and very little protein? | ✓ | ✓ | ✓ | |

| | HORMONAL IMBALANCE | BLOOD-SUGAR | INFLAMMATION | AGING |
|---|---|---|---|---|
| Do you have aches and pains or sore joints? | | | ✓ | ✓ |
| Do you experience digestive problems such as bloating, reflux, ulcers, or food sensitivities? | | | ✓ | |
| Do you feel chronically stressed? | | | ✓ | |
| Do you often drink more than 4 alcoholic drinks in one week? | | | ✓ | ✓ |
| Are you a smoker? | | | ✓ | ✓ |
| Do you have sinus congestion, hayfever or asthma? | | | ✓ | |
| Are you over 35 if you're a woman or over 40 if you're a man? | | | | ✓ |
| Do you eat any of these foods on most days of the week: red meat, fried or processed foods (e.g. packaged foods, biscuits etc), sugar, white bread, cakes, soft drinks? | ✓ | ✓ | ✓ | ✓ |
| Do you eat less than or 3 cups of veggies and 2 fruits a day? | | | ✓ | ✓ |

| | HORMONAL IMBALANCE | BLOOD-SUGAR | INFLAMMATION | AGING |
|---|---|---|---|---|
| Have you been diagnosed with an auto-immune condition or auto-immune antibodies? | | | ✓ | |
| Have you experienced recurrent pregnancy loss? | ✓ | | ✓ | ✓ |
| Are you undergoing IVF or been advised you have egg quality issues? | ✓ | ✓ | ✓ | ✓ |
| SCORE | | | | |

**SCORE:** 1 or more 'ticks'

If you highlighted or circled any of these questions, then to get the most from this book please read the recommended chapter in Part 3 Your health, hormones and fertility. The most relevant for you will be the columns you had the most responses in. For example, if it was the "hormonal imbalance" column then turn to Part 3: Chapter 13.

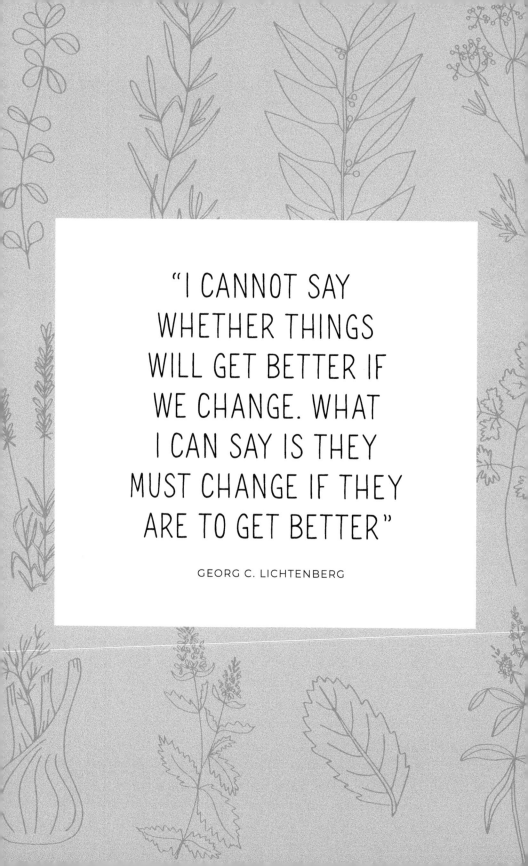

"I CANNOT SAY WHETHER THINGS WILL GET BETTER IF WE CHANGE. WHAT I CAN SAY IS THEY MUST CHANGE IF THEY ARE TO GET BETTER"

GEORG C. LICHTENBERG

# PART ONE

# Plant the Seeds
## The essential guide to improving your fertility

# IN THIS SECTION:

# 1

# Your health team

Getting a health team together sooner rather than later can assist you in conceiving more consciously, with greater confidence while knowing you are doing the best for your own health and that of your baby and future family. Choose experienced professionals you can trust. Whether you are just starting to think about making a family, are trying to conceive now or already know you have fertility challenges, they will be there to support you and help you map your way through. A good supportive team with varying points of view can help ensure that potential problems are identified and treated, and nothing gets missed. This is true holistic health care.

Your health team will help you identify and understand any challenges you face and what you can do to overcome them or improve your potential. Learning how to be and stay healthy, how to optimise your fertility and feeling supported in making necessary changes can not only make the path less daunting and less stressful but will also maximise your chances of conceiving. You don't know what you don't know, so a team of helpful professionals will ensure you get your needs met and give you the confidence to make a realistic and effective plan for your fertility.

In an ideal world we would recommend getting a team in place a minimum of four months before trying to conceive. That way you will have support to inspire you to prepare your health and your body for conception and pregnancy. In the real world just start when you can wherever you are on your conception path. If you haven't already, start now.

## TEAM COLLABORATION

Ideally your whole team will be open to communication in all directions. This ensures everyone is informed about what is going on and has the relevant information to provide you with the best possible care. Good complementary health practitioners will write to your GP and/or specialist (with your permission) to keep them informed about treatment. There are times when something we prescribe may have implications for them. It also ensures that if they have any concerns they can be in contact with us to check in. Collaboration between practitioners (naturopaths, acupuncturists, GPs and specialists) really ups the safety element and we believe ensures the best care for our patients. Your medical practitioner may not communicate with natural health practitioners as a standard part of their practice, so if they don't have an existing relationship with your other practitioners, please do ask that they copy them in on any correspondence they are sending to their medical colleagues and ensure they send copies of all tests at the time of testing. Of course, the same goes both ways for your natural medicine practitioners.

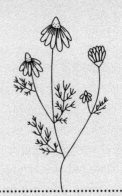

# It really helps to know your test results

**Please keep copies of all your test results in chronological order including ultrasounds, blood tests and any other tests you have done. Ask any previous doctors or specialists for copies of relevant test results or procedure summaries as these will paint a clear picture of your health history. We recommend that you take this file along to all your appointments. By becoming informed and taking an active role in your health, you will already be making steps along the right path and be in a much better position to learn and add more benefit from your health team.**

## FIND A GOOD GENERAL PRACTITIONER (GP)

Finding a GP you are comfortable with and who is willing to do some good pre-conception tests is a great place to start. They are likely to do some routine screening checks including measles, mumps, rubella (German measles) and varicella (chickenpox), hepatitis B and C, HIV and syphilis. It is important to know your blood group and make sure your pap smear testing and breast exams are up to date before you are pregnant as well. Ensure that you communicate any other health concerns and discuss the safety of any medication you may be taking (prescribed or otherwise) at this stage, so that appropriate investigation, action or advice may be carried out before you conceive.

# WHAT WILL A NATUROPATH DO TO ENHANCE A HEALTHY CONCEPTION?

We recommend employing the support of a qualified and experienced fertility naturopath for everyone wishing to conceive. Naturopaths will help couples optimise their health prior to conception and ensure they have the healthiest pregnancy possible, and best health outcomes for both mother and child. Naturopaths also work to assist, treat and support couples and individuals with diagnosed fertility issues or those having trouble conceiving.

Supporting your pre-conception health and pregnancy with good food and nutrition is the first important step. There is so much research now indicating the importance of both potential parents' nutritional health in the months prior to conception affecting the long-term health of the offspring. Getting some professional input at this early stage has huge benefits. Alongside nutrition and diet advice, adequate sunshine, rest, sleep, and regular moderate exercise will all be assessed. A good naturopath will guide you through charting your cycle and identifying your fertile window for conception, ensure appropriate testing has been carried out with your GP and they will also discuss how to reduce your environmental toxin exposure.

If you find a naturopath who is experienced in treating both men and women with fertility issues, as well as pregnancy support, then they can provide you with a wealth of information.

Your experienced naturopath can help you determine which supplements are the best quality, what doses are relevant for you at this stage of your fertility journey and when to take them and stop them. Some supplements will be advisable to continue in pregnancy and others not. For example, some herbs are safe in pregnancy and others are best avoided. We generally recommend no herbal medicine unless prescribed by your qualified and experienced naturopath/

herbalist. Some herbs may also interact with medications. This is particularly so if you are undergoing IVF or other hormonal treatment.

Along with general conception preparation, naturopaths will take a detailed case history about your reproductive and general health and may be able to immediately assess a number of areas where they can boost your fertility. They will work with you towards hormonal balance, optimising your cycle and reproductive health, address other acute or chronic health concerns and ensure good nutrition and supplementation for crucial nutrient levels. This work gives the starting cells that will make your baby – your eggs and sperm – all they need for optimal health and function. It is a vital part of any treatment plan for a couple or individual trying to conceive.

# WHY NOT PICK-UP THE SUPPLEMENTS I NEED FROM A HEALTH FOOD STORE?

You will notice in this book we have not listed many supplements as a general rule. That's because it's not the same for everyone and you need advice from someone who knows your full health history and other particulars to ensure the right supplements to take, how much, how often, for how long and when to stop. Plus, not all supplements are created equal. Do you know why one fish oil is better than another? What are the levels of the EPA and DHA in your fish oils and have they been tested for mercury levels? Have they been processed with peroxide and damaged? While we often recommend a quality fish oil and a natal multivitamin/mineral ideally with good levels of well-absorbed nutrients, deciding on which ones to use is complex. So please take our advice and find an experienced naturopath or nutritionist as poor-quality supplements, taking the wrong doses or taking the wrong supplement entirely can be a waste of time and money or indeed do more harm than good.

# WHEN DOES ACUPUNCTURE AND TRADITIONAL CHINESE MEDICINE (TCM) COME INTO IT?

TCM and naturopathic approaches are highly compatible and commonly combined in patients with fertility challenges for optimum results.

When you see a TCM practitioner or acupuncturist for a consultation, they will commonly feel your pulse at your wrists and look at your tongue, face and possibly palpate along acupuncture channels (meridians) in your body where appropriate. Combined with a full case history, TCM practitioners determine where the energy is deficient or too full in any particular channels. Along with very effective needling techniques and possibly herbs to correct any imbalance found in any energy channels, they can use certain points to improve the functioning of your ovaries and testicles (don't worry, the points are not on the testicles!!) and directly affect the quality of the developing eggs and sperm. Sometimes they employ other techniques such as moxibustion (applying heat to the points), laser or electro acupuncture, or cupping and massage too, depending on what is required for your individual needs, TCM diagnosis and health goals.

Perhaps the best thing about acupuncture is that you get to stop, lie down and relax for a good half hour or more. In our practice you are made warm and toasty with blankets and wheat bags, you have eye pillows and headphones and our practitioners play our guided meditations (or music if you prefer) so you get the ultimate relaxation experience.

Your practitioner will also talk with you about your diet and lifestyle from the perspective that may be causing any imbalance, and suggest practical solutions you can work on at home. While ultimately working toward the same outcomes, you can see that TCM practitioners and naturopaths address the issues from very different angles. In our experience, it gets patients to their goals more quickly and in a more holistic way, taking all possibilities into consideration.

Although the understanding of acupuncture is based on an ancient medical theory, thousands of years old, the body of research-based evidence on Chinese herbal medicine and acupuncture for fertility is growing.

For Chinese herbal medicine, a meta-analysis of quality research articles suggested that herbal management of female infertility can improve pregnancy rates two-fold within a three to six-month period compared with Western medical fertility drug therapy or IVF. Fertility indicators such as ovulation rates, cervical mucus score, basal body temperature ovulation indicators, and appropriate thickness of the endometrial lining were positively influenced by Chinese herbal medicine, indicating physiological improvements that will support a viable pregnancy.[15]

Another systematic review comparing Chinese herbal medicine to the medication clomiphine (Clomid), prescribed for women who do not ovulate (anovulation), showed that the herbs had better outcomes for improving ovulation and cervical mucus scores as well as positive pregnancy and reducing miscarriage rates, with no significant adverse effects for the herbal medicine groups.[16]

Assessment of the quality of the menstrual cycle, integral to TCM diagnosis, appears to be fundamental to successful treatment of female infertility, highlighting the importance of an individual approach - there is no "one size fits all" or standard protocols when it comes to natural medicine.

There is much more that Chinese medicine and acupuncture has to offer people with fertility problems and there is some research to suggest it has the following reproductive effects.

## Acupuncture for women

o Support egg development by regulating hormones and ovulation.[17]

o Influences hormonal action and menstrual cycle regulation via endogenous opioids (endorphins) impacting on the hypothalamic-pituitary-ovarian axis[18]

o Improves physical and psychological symptoms of premenstrual syndrome[19]

o Helps improve the ovarian response to hormonal stimulation (including IVF).[20]

o Helps reduce FSH levels, important if you are in early or near peri-menopause.[21]

o Helps support implantation by improving blood flow to a woman's pelvic area and the uterus.[18,22,23]

o Helps to improve endometrial receptivity.[23]

o Helps reduce pelvic cramping and period pain,[24] as well as inflammation modulation.[25]

## Acupuncture for men

o Helps improve sperm motility, morphology (shape) and count.[26,27]

## For both men and women

o Helps to relax and reduce the impact of stress on the reproductive system.[28,29]

# BONUS — YOU WILL FEEL BETTER TOO

As you can see, a natural medicine team will look at your overall health and not just your reproductive history. This is essential for a comprehensive approach to your fertility. Patients are often surprised about how good they feel after a few weeks or months of treatment, and of course we hope they may also have conceived and be on the way to a healthy baby.

# OTHER PROFESSIONAL SUPPORT

You may need to look to others to help you with particular health goals. Maybe a skilled counsellor, osteopath, massage therapist or a personal trainer would be a good person to add to your team.

For example, if trying to conceive is taking longer than you thought or you are coming across challenges you weren't expecting with your fertility or perhaps your relationship, then finding a counsellor or psychologist you can work with is an integral part of a team to keep you mentally well, your partnership, family and friend relationships intact, help you manage stress and to help build emotional resilience around any treatment.

Osteopathy can ensure your nervous system and blood flow is adequately supplying your reproductive area from a structural point of view, and prepare your body for when you are pregnant and carrying a heavy load. If you experience regular pelvic or lower back or abdominal pain, an osteopathic assessment is highly recommended.

Massage is a wonderful part of a relaxation strategy and could be included as regularly as you like. It is particularly great to enjoy a massage at the most stressful parts of your cycle if you are trying to conceive — around ovulation time to help you feel relaxed and receptive, and towards the end of the cycle when you may be feeling anxious about getting your period. Once you have established that your massage therapist is experienced and understands the potential contra-indications for massage in pregnancy, ask if they know of any fertility massage techniques to help improve blood flow to the reproductive area. This is commonly performed as abdominal massage. Some people also find reflexology to be beneficial, and while there is no research to support it, who wouldn't love a regular foot massage!

## WHAT FURTHER MEDICAL TESTS TO CONSIDER IF YOU HAVEN'T CONCEIVED?

If you have been trying for 6-12 months without a positive pregnancy test, then your doctor may recommend more thorough testing. This may start with some hormonal blood tests to check ovulation, an ultrasound to check the health of your ovaries and uterus, and a semen analysis. The male investigation (semen analysis) is often overlooked and is well worth asking for at this stage. If you are over 35 and have been trying for six months or more, we recommend that you request more thorough investigations simply because these tests might take some time. At this stage the doctor may refer you to a gynaecologist or fertility specialist. If you do need assisted reproduction, as statistical success rates do drop with age, it is a good idea not to wait too long before seeking further investigations.

## WHEN SHOULD WE FAST-TRACK TO ASSISTED REPRODUCTIVE TECHNOLOGY (ART)?

Whether to go to assisted reproduction and/or IVF will be a decision you and your partner need to discuss. If this is something you would consider, please do ensure that a reliable sperm test has been performed (ideally at an IVF or andrology laboratory) before undergoing the many potential (and often much more invasive) female investigations. It is also worth asking about checking your ovarian reserve at this stage for an indication of how many eggs you have left, especially if you are 35 or over and have been trying for six months or more. If it is low for your age, then you may want to consider going straight to see a fertility specialist and assess your medical treatment options. Having the rest of your team in place at this stage (naturopath, GP, acupuncturist) will ensure you get comprehensive advice and good interventions early.

Take a deep breath. A referral to a fertility specialist doesn't signal disaster. Even if something is found to be an issue, often a diagnosis can give direction where you have had none. Not everyone will get a definitive diagnosis, and in our experience many couples have complex issues often affecting them both. The medical approach has some good things to offer, especially in the way of surgical interventions if necessary and, of course, in the IVF process itself. However, there are some clear gaps, especially when it comes to optimising your chances and recovery after any surgical intervention. A combined approach ensures you have all the bases covered. Many fertility specialists are now seeing the benefits for their patients and enjoying collaborating with us.

## DO YOU NEED A NATUROPATH AND ACUPUNCTURIST IF YOU ARE UNDERGOING ART OR IVF?

Increasingly, many of our local IVF specialists have found the benefit for their clients seeing a naturopath and acupuncturist at the same time as undergoing IVF. The healthier the couples are the better the chances of successful IVF – and some of our patients are even able to conceive naturally between IVF cycles!

# Mandy's Story

41-year-old Mandy consulted the clinic after being referred by an existing patient. At the time, she had been trying to conceive for six months and all testing had indicated there were no other fertility issues apart from the impact of her age on egg quality.

Mandy and her partner had undergone four unsuccessful IVF cycles. Each IVF cycle had similar results with six eggs being retrieved at egg collection and only two of these fertilising. All embryo transfers had been unsuccessful.

Mandy was also on medication for hypothyroidism and had blood tests indicating she was low in a number of nutrients (including iron and vitamin D), had slightly high cholesterol, and her thyroid function was less than optimal. As Mandy was preparing for her fifth IVF cycle, an appropriate preconception time to focus on improving egg quality was discussed. This included taking supplements, making some changes to her diet (primarily cutting out all alcohol, coffee, increasing her water and fish intake) and starting regular exercise and acupuncture.

At her next round of blood tests a few months later, all her nutrients levels had improved, and both her cholesterol and thyroid function had normalised (the latter occurred even without a change in her thyroid medication). Overall, her health was much better.

Mandy then proceeded with her IVF cycle, which resulted in not only more eggs retrieved (eight eggs) and better fertilisation rates (six fertilised), it is also resulted in a positive pregnancy and a beautiful baby girl.

If you do need IVF to help you conceive, attending to as many of the factors of good preconception health care outlined throughout this book will ensure you have the best chance of successful outcomes. You will see so much evidence supporting diet and lifestyle modification throughout the coming pages and it is equally if not more important for IVF to do what you can. Egg and sperm quality is of paramount importance now, as is the lining of the uterus for implantation and we can make a real difference here. Embryologists we work with say they can see the difference in the embryos they create when people start taking specific nutrients and change their diet and lifestyle and fertility specialists say the can see a difference in the quality of the endometrial lining too. Side-effects like bloating, fluid retention and pain are minimised with these complementary approaches, and the nervous system and adrenals are adequately supported.

Fertility specialists who we work with also comment on the fabulous benefits of stress reduction techniques, and nutrients and herbs prescribed to support the nervous system when their patients are going through IVF. With all this support, these couples and individuals are more able to cope with the ups and downs of their IVF treatment. Rather than a downward spiral in health due to the stress of IVF and the side effects of treatment, most of our patients feel much better for working positively on their health and feel empowered that there are things they can do that can make a real difference.

There is a wealth of scientific evidence to support our naturopathic guidelines for preconception health care and the best outcomes for creating your healthy baby – regardless of if you are trying to conceive naturally or with ART/IVF. Read on through the rest of the book to find out more!

Importantly, never self-prescribe herbs, nutrients or other things you may read about being helpful for IVF on the internet (or are recommended by "helpful" friends) while you are doing IVF. The herb/nutrient-drug reactions can be problematic and even dangerous in some cases.[30-32] Please seek the advice of a qualified fertility naturopath to work out the best plan for you that will support your aims. It is too important to mess around with "trying" things out.

Interestingly, a large proportion of the research on acupuncture for fertility is focused on the impact of acupuncture during IVF treatment. The most recent Australian review of all of the English-speaking evidence published in 2019 is clear and positive.[18]

o Acupuncture with IVF may have potentially significant benefits when compared to IVF only, in regard to both clinical pregnancy AND live birth rates.

o Acupuncture seems most effective when there are more treatments (higher dose), especially with a treatment in the stimulation, day of transfer and implantation phase.

o Further benefits are seen when points selected are tailored to the individual rather than using a pre-prescribed treatment protocol.

o Benefits are especially true for women who have had multiple previous IVF cycles.

o Acupuncture may be working via the stress relieving and psychosocial benefits with a significant anxiolytic effect reported and potential beneficial effects such as increase in uterine blood flow (for a healthy uterine lining), endogenous endorphins (natural pain relief and happy feelings) and cytokines (regulate immune function, inflammation and even reproduction to some degree).

o   The research review also discusses the benefits of the holistic nature of the consultation process too - with palpation, education, self-care and diagnosis all cited as helpful components of the treatment process.

o   Finally acupuncture is a low risk intervention that women undergoing IVF should know about.

Some evidence over the years has been focused on the benefits of just two treatments on the day of embryo transfer – generally known as pre and post transfer acupuncture. While undoubtedly this will have some benefit (blood flow to the pelvic area, calming the uterine environment and supported relaxation for the anxiety of what can otherwise be a pretty busy and stressful day), this is not a sufficient dose of acupuncture for improving outcomes in pregnancy and birth and not considered to be effective for this.[33,34]

Higher dose acupuncture weekly for the whole stimulated IVF cycle, and where possible, weekly in the 2-3 cycles leading up to the IVF cycle will give much better results. This is backed up by a number of systematic reviews and a retrospective study that analysed results of more that 1000 IVF cycles, finding that 9-12 treatments prior to embryo transfer was associated with more live births.[35,36] It also showed that the best outcomes were for those women receiving whole-system traditional Chinese medicine, which may include individualised Chinese herbal medicine, dietary and lifestyle recommendations. The whole-system TCM group had a live birth rate of 61.3% compared to 48.2% in the IVF only group and 50.8% in the group having acupuncture only on day of embryo transfer.[20] It makes total sense when considering that acupuncture in the three months before an IVF cycle is going to impact the environment while the eggs are maturing, and this increased dosing of acupuncture has the more significant effect.

# How often do I need acupuncture for my best chances in IVF?

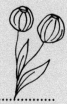

**We recommend weekly appointments in the two to three cycles (months) leading up to IVF.**

**When your IVF cycle starts (or if you have already started) then your acupuncturist may recommend more frequent treatments to help support optimal outcomes. At least once before the transfer as the follicles are being medically stimulated, one to two times on the day of transfer, and another treatment around five to seven days after transfer for implantation support.**

**Wherever you are at in your IVF cycle or if you are planning for IVF, start now! See a fertility acupuncturist ASAP to work out the best plan for you.**

Clinically we find that this holistic approach encompassing individual care and whole-system Chinese medicine with adequate dosing of acupuncture, allowing longer term treatment, is more effective.

While it is so good to read this scientific validation of the use of acupuncture and Chinese herbal medicine[37] in conjunction with IVF, for us, although our patients having a take home baby is obviously a key desired outcome, benefits of treatment are not only about the pregnancy and live birth rates. Reduced anxiety levels and a better ability to cope with infertility and IVF is so important for people with poor outcomes, fragile emotional health, and those doing back to back cycles who need to 'gear up again' after a negative result. This effect cannot be underestimated (and there is even some research to support this too[38-40]). Sometimes it can be the difference between patients feeling like they have the internal resources to take on the next cycle, or need a break. Regular acupuncture with practitioners skilled in working with IVF patients can provide support they need to navigate their experience as seamlessly as possible, potentially with fewer side effects and positive outcomes more quickly.

# ONCE YOU ARE PREGNANT

Once you fall pregnant either naturally or through assisted reproduction, it is important to continue consulting with your team. You'll be adding new people to your team too - a midwife team or one to one midwife at a public hospital, a private independent midwife or an obstetrician and even a doula or birth attendant. Ask your current team who they recommend and collaborate well with to continue best care and positive outcomes.

For every pregnant woman, your nutritional needs during pregnancy and breastfeeding are the highest you will experience in your life. And with a developing baby on board it is important to get it right. Your practitioners will focus on:

o   Optimising your health and baby's health, growth and development needs.

o   Reducing your risk of miscarriage.

o   Nutritional support (what you should/shouldn't be eating plus appropriate supplementation).

o   Safely treating any pregnancy-related conditions such as nausea, vomiting, cramping, constipation and more.

o   Reducing your risk of pregnancy complications such as gestational diabetes.

o   Labour and birth preparation to help reduce your risk of interventions and prepare for a positive, empowering birth experience.

o   Preparation for breastfeeding.

# TOP TIPS FOR HER

Consider a process of three to four months
of preconception care if time is on your side.

Ask your GP for routine pre-conception blood tests. Keep all
test results in your own file and take to all appointments.

Surround yourself with an experienced team. Include at
least a GP, naturopath and/or acupuncturist (experienced
in support of fertility and/or IVF). Consider what other
support or resources you might need, like massage,
personal training, osteopathic care etc.

If you are under 35 years old and haven't conceived within
a year, seek further help. If you are over 35 years old, seek
help after six months. Always seek help early if either
yourself or your partner has a history of any conditions
known to impact fertility e.g. endometriosis, PCOS,
history of undescended testes etc.

If you are unsure about advice you have been given,
check with your health team, or get a second opinion.

If you are having further investigations and it's
taking longer than you thought to conceive,
consider seeing a counsellor to help with any
feelings that may arise related to your
fertility challenges.

# TOP TIPS FOR HIM

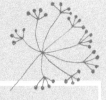

Consider a process of three to four months
of preconception care if time is on your side.

Get routine pre-conception blood tests from your GP. Keep
all test results in your own file and take to all appointments.

Ensure your sperm is tested early in the process (preferably
at an IVF lab) if conception does not happen easily – within
12 months if your partner is under 35 years old, or within
six months if your partner is 35 years old or over.

Always seek help early if either yourself or your partner
has a history of any conditions known to impact fertility
e.g. undescended testes, endometriosis, PCOS etc.

If sperm issues are part of the problem, get on to an
experienced naturopath ASAP. Your naturopath may
recommend further testing to determine underlying issues
contributing to sperm problems, and will recommend
nutritional and herbal approaches to improve your fertility.

If you are needing further investigations and it's taking longer
than you thought to conceive consider seeing a counsellor to
help with any feelings that may arise related to your fertility
challenges. Many men find talking about their reproductive
health embarrassing or demeaning. A counsellor can
provide support and information, help you to develop coping
strategies and a different perspective on your situation.

# 2

# Sex and timing:
# let's talk about sex

It can be so easy to get caught up in the dos and don'ts of trying to conceive – don't drink alcohol, go to your GP for testing, give up the cigarettes, exercise more – that we can forget to talk about the most important thing about getting pregnant: SEX!

When you first start consciously trying to conceive, sex with your partner may be the most potent love-making you have experienced. To come together to make a baby is ultimately what it is all about – a culmination of your love together resulting in the formation of another human being whose every cell is made up of your union. Amazing times!

But it seems that it can quickly turn to stressful thinking, especially as we often assume that it will happen quickly and easily for us. We have tried so hard for most of our reproductive lives to not get pregnant with intercourse, it is easy to assume that it should happen on the first attempt without contraception. Right?

# HOW LONG WILL IT TAKE TO CONCEIVE?

We know that around 80-84% of couples with healthy and fully-functioning reproductive systems will be pregnant within 12 months, and 93% within two years.[41,42] These couples have a 20% chance of conceiving on any one cycle and the chance is not cumulative – it is a 20% chance each time.[43,44] We also know that a variety of factors can affect your chance of conceiving, including your age, diet, lifestyle, fitness and stress levels.[45] We will get to all of that, but let's focus on sex first!

---

**A fertility equation**

If 100 couples try to get pregnant in January, about 20 will conceive, leaving 80 to try again in February. If another 20 per cent (or 16 couples) conceive, then 64 will be trying again in March. Continuing the one-in-five success rate, by the end of April roughly half will have successfully conceived. At this rate, after seven months 78 couples would have conceived (leaving 22 not yet pregnant).

---

Trying to conceive (TTC) takes time – it is like predicting the weather really. It can look like rain, feel like rain, even have lightning and thunder and yet still hold off. It will rain eventually in most cases, but we can't say exactly when. When you start TTC, if you can, try to keep hold of the understanding that you would like to conceive sometime over the course of the year. This will help avoid what many couples experience as the roller-coaster ride of TTC – the highs and lows that come with expectation and disappointment if you don't have a positive pregnancy test; feelings that are often compounded by PMT!

Having said that though, research shows that if you can interpret your body's signs of ovulation and time your sex and conception attempts to the fertile window, your chances of conceiving on any one cycle are significantly higher.[46]

## SO WHEN IS THE BEST TIME TO HAVE SEX?

Every pregnancy truly is a miracle of its own. When it comes to getting pregnant, it seems that many couples aren't doing it right. A recent Australian study of women trying to conceive found that although more than half (68.2%) thought they were timing it right for conception, only 13% accurately estimated their day of ovulation.[9]

Understanding the most fertile time of the female cycle is critical for conception to occur and it is so important to get good education and advice about this.[47] An inaccurate understanding may contribute to delayed conception and many cases of 'unexplained' infertility. Women only have a small window in each reproductive cycle to conceive so it is important to get the timing right. While you can feel like you have been trying for months and months, if you are not focusing your efforts on this optimal window of time, the likelihood of conceiving is slim.

## Jane's Story

*Jane had been trying to conceive based on when her app told her she was 'flowering'. Sure enough, as her cycle was irregular (31-45 days), it was way off, saying that she was ovulating a lot earlier than she was and hence missing the fertile window for healthy conception. This couple tried the next month at the right time, and low and behold it worked! Jane also made diet changes and had started herbal medicine, but the timing was an important factor.*

# THE FERTILE WINDOW

We know that eggs only live for 12-24 hours while sperm may be viable for up to five days (although most have very little vitality left after three).[1] For optimal chances and the healthiest conception, ideally sperm will be ready and waiting in the fallopian tubes for when the egg is released by the ovary (ovulation). The best chances of conceiving occur with intercourse within the two days before ovulation and the day of ovulation.[46] These three days are called your 'Fertile Window'.

Technically, you do have a small chance of conception from five days prior to ovulation but you have the highest probability during this three-day window. This is also the best time for insemination for same-sex couples or single women who are planning to time insemination at home. In most cases you don't need to rely on technology or your doctor to tell you when this is occurring. Happily, there are signs to indicate the fertile window and that the egg is about to be released.

### When is my fertile window?

To improve your chances of conception, have sex during the two days prior to ovulation and the day of ovulation. e.g if you ovulate on Day 14 of your cycle, your most fertile days (and also the best to have sex) are likely to be days 12, 13 and 14.

Having said that, ovulation can be affected by many factors – stress, weight (over and under), excessive exercise, excitement, travel, thyroid problems, polycystic ovarian syndrome and anaemia (as well as all the various types of infertility). Read on for more information on how you can understand how to determine your fertile window, but it is important to seek guidance with a qualified and experienced fertility professional if you are confused.

# HOW DO I KNOW WHEN I OVULATE TO DETERMINE MY FERTILE WINDOW?

Where time permits, it is useful to check and record the signs and symptoms of your reproductive cycle for a few cycles before you try to conceive. In Appendix 2, we have included the chart you will need, and a link to download the full sized version from our website. Print it out to keep by your bedside table and record your signs and symptoms daily. To understand how to use this chart, read below.

Knowing your signs of ovulation and timing your sex with understanding of your cycle will give you an increased sense of confidence in your conscious conception. Marking secondary symptoms like headaches or fluid retention will give your fertility practitioner team very useful information about your cycle and hormones to assist with providing the best treatment for your individual needs.

Make sure you scan and email or bring your charts to every fertility-related appointment where possible. Your practitioner will help you to understand and interpret your chart with ease. It may seem confusing at first, but within a few cycles it will become clear – a free and easy method to understand your cycle for your reproductive life.

## 1. TRACKING YOUR CYCLE LENGTH

Tracking the days of your cycle to work out when you ovulate is otherwise known as the rhythm method, and the main method used by many fertility apps.

Cycle tracking is an important part of understanding your fertility and this information will evolve as you chart the details of your cycle. It is important to know, however, that timing your conception attempts to the rhythm method or fertility apps is only possible if you have a very regular cycle. Ovulation generally occurs 14 days before your period (not on Day 14 as is commonly misunderstood). You need to know when to expect your period so you can work backwards.

Remembering the three-day optimal fertile window, look back on your last few cycles and count the days. Day 1 of your cycle is the first day of your menstrual flow (not spotting) and the last day of your cycle is the last day before your next flow. If you regularly have a 28 day cycle, ovulation will generally occur at Day 14 so your fertile window starts at Day 12. If you have shorter cycles of around 21 days, your ovulation will likely occur at Day 7 so your fertile window starts at Day 5. If you have a longer cycle of around 35 days, you will generally ovulate on Day 21 so your fertile window starts at Day 19.

Having said that, it is possible to have a shorter luteal phase (ovulation to menstruation) or irregular cycles, and this can confuse timing. It is common in these instances to have other signs of menstrual function disturbance such as little or no fertile mucus, a variety of premenstrual symptoms including mood changes, tiredness, skin eruptions or cramping, spotting mid-cycle or before your menstrual flow, or period pain. If this is the case, you don't need to suffer! A qualified and experienced naturopath or Chinese medicine practitioner may assist with herbal medicine, acupuncture or addressing underlying nutritional or lifestyle imbalances to improve cycle regulation, follicular and egg development and hormonal balance.

So whilst the rhythm method or fertility apps can be helpful with regard to timing if your cycle is regular, it can be quite inaccurate if your cycle varies in length.

## 2. KNOW YOUR SECRETIONS

For most of your cycle, your cervix produces a mucus barrier to sperm – almost like a plug, with a thick white mucus that blocks the entry to the womb both physically (as a barrier) and chemically (with immune components that fight foreign materials). We refer to this mucus as 'infertile' mucus and it is normal to have this type of mucus at various stages of your cycle (mostly just before and just after your period). As the follicles grow in readiness for ovulation, the balance of hormones produced enable a change in the cervical mucus to facilitate the passage of the sperm towards the egg. The mucus secretions become noticeably wetter and more stretchy and slippery in the days leading up to ovulation, with peak symptoms occurring just before the egg is released. At a microscopic level, the mucus is actually forming channels for the sperm to swim through, as well as providing nourishment for the journey of healthy sperm, and a quality control system to remove damaged or dysfunctional sperm.

Many women also report an increase in libido at this time – more evolutionary genius to further the continuation of the species!

Where time permits, it is useful to check and record the signs and symptoms of your cycle for a few cycles before you try to conceive. Knowing your signs of ovulation and timing your sex with ease will give you an increased sense of confidence in your conscious conception and improve your chances of conception.[48]

## Checking and recording your cervical mucus changes

Check your mucus each time you go to the toilet, before urination, by wiping at the opening to your vagina or inserting your finger about 1-2 cm into the vagina and then stretching the mucus out between two fingers. Record the amount, colour, texture and external sensation on your chart. Develop a consistent code that works for you over time to make recording easy and readable. Always record the most fertile mucus (the most wet, watery, slimy, slippery or stretchy mucus) you noticed that day.

o   Your basic infertile pattern of mucus can vary from none/dry or damp, pasty, flaky, crumbly, thick or dense in the non-fertile phases. As ovulation approaches, the mucus pattern will change to creamy or milky and start to become wetter. Your fertile mucus will be clear, wet, watery, slimy, slippery or stretchy at ovulation, more like egg white.

o   How does the outside of your vagina feel? Is it wet or dry, moist or damp? The wetter the sensation, the more fertile you are.

o   The amount of mucus will increase the closer you get to ovulation. Is there a lot of it, a medium amount, or very little?

o   Each woman is different, and mucus can vary from one cycle to another, although generally an obvious pattern will emerge for you. After a couple of cycles are charted, you may start to notice that ovulation generally occurs four days after your mucus changes from your basic infertile pattern to a wetter and more slippery mucus. Or perhaps you have three days of pasty mucus followed by one day of egg white. What is it for you?

o   Immediately after ovulation, there is a marked decrease in mucus production, with a quick return to your basic infertile pattern. You can confirm ovulation has occurred if you are charting your temperature as well (see below), or via a blood test seven days later (the Day 21 progesterone test).

o   Understanding your mucus pattern is the best way to identify approaching ovulation and getting the timing right for sex and conception, as temperature charting and the rhythm method will only confirm that ovulation has already occurred, and you will miss the fertile window time.

o   It can be very helpful to talk to an expert in fertility charting to understand your mucus pattern.

| PHASE | SENSATION | CERVICAL MUCUS APPEARANCE |
|---|---|---|
| Infertile | Dry | No visible mucus. |
| Ovulation approaching | Moist or sticky | White or cream-coloured, thick to slightly stretchy. Breaks easily when stretched. |
| Highly Fertile | Slippery, wet, lubricated | Increase in amount. Thin, stretchy, watery, transparent, like egg white. |
| After ovulation infertile | Dry or sticky | Sharp decrease in amount. Thick, opaque-white or cream-coloured. |

It can be difficult to detect cervical mucus after sex due to the presence of semen, and your mucus can also be altered by infection and some medications. When cervical secretions are reduced in quantity or quality it may be associated with an underlying hormonal imbalance or issues with follicular development, egg quality or health of the cervix. Thus, it is important to address these issues. Your experienced naturopath or Chinese medicine practitioner will be able to help you here.

When you know your ovulation signs you can ensure that you are getting the timing right with sex the day or two before and on the day of ovulation when the mucus is at its most fertile. Sex within this fertile window dramatically improves your chances of conceiving compared with untimed frequent sex throughout the cycle.

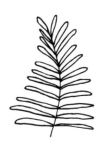

## Should he restrain from ejaculation to build up the sperm?

..........................................................................................................

Some research has shown that sperm quality is improved with frequent ejaculation. It seems that daily ejaculation may reduce the amount of DNA damage that sperm would otherwise suffer if stored for too long before a conception attempt.[49-51] While ejaculate volume may reduce a little, the sperm contained seem to benefit with improved DNA, and even improvements to motility so it is recommended for a healthier conception.

Based on this research it seems that it may help having sex daily or every second day in the three days leading up to and on the day of ovulation. Keep in mind that from a Chinese medicine perspective it is thought that frequent ejaculation may reduce sexual energy and adversely impact on reproductive health. So don't focus on this. Instead, have sex depending on your energy levels and sex drive.

## 3. TEST YOUR URINE TO DETECT WHEN YOU MAY BE APPROACHING OVULATION

Ovulation Predictor Kits (OPKs) can be useful as they test for a surge in Luteinising Hormone (LH) – the hormone that initiates the release of the egg. Tracking your mucus changes is usually sufficient to indicate impending ovulation. However, if you want extra information then OPKs are a simple (albeit pricey) test (available online or at a supermarket or chemist) that you begin three days before you anticipate your ovulation (i.e. subtract 17 days from your expected menstruation date). Start earlier if you are unsure when this is, or follow the guidelines on your kit. Ovulation usually occurs 24-36 hours after a positive result, so it is ideal to have sex as soon as you see a positive result). It is important to note however, that a positive result does not guarantee ovulation will occur, which leads us to...

# 4. CHART YOUR TEMPERATURE

Many women are confused about the value of temperature taking when trying to conceive. There are a lot of arguments for and against charting, and many medical fertility specialists seem to agree that it is more stressful than useful so best not to bother at all. However, charting your temperature can provide a lot of useful information to someone who knows how to interpret it, and once you have had your unique pattern of temperature explained, it is actually quite easy to understand and can be incredibly empowering!

It is important to take your temperature first thing in the morning with a digital thermometer under the tongue. When we say first thing, we mean before you talk to your partner, sip on a cup of tea or even move much – you wake up, roll over and put your thermometer in your mouth and wait until it beeps. Many thermometers keep the temperature displayed until you use it again, so you don't have to record it straight away if it is still dark or you are trying not to wake your partner.

Usually, there will be a 'thermal shift' (temperature increase) of about ½ a degree Celsius that indicates ovulation has occurred. The temperature starts to shift after the egg is released – the rule is three over five – you need to see three mornings of higher temperatures than the last five. This is why you can't use temperature charts to time your conception attempts, as once the shift has occurred, ovulation is already over and you have missed your chance.

You can, however, record any sex you have had and use your chart to see if you did indeed get the timing right in that cycle to know that you are in with a chance.

# Should I wait until my temperature rises before having sex?

Having sex on the day your temperature rises does not increase your chances of conception – in fact it may decrease your chances. As the egg is only viable for 12-24 hours, chances are you will miss the opportunity. If you wait until the 'thermal shift' to have sex you may have missed your most fertile time. Charting is used to help you know your pattern so you can pre-empt the rise with mucus changes and ensure you have sex at the right time.

## Checking and recording your resting temperature

o You need an ovulation or digital thermometer designed for under the tongue use. Do not use an ear thermometer.

o Have the thermometer beside your bed before you go to sleep. On waking, before getting out of bed or even talking, take your temperature by placing the thermometer under your tongue. It is important to make as little movement as possible whilst taking your temperature to get a true resting temperature. Place a dot in the box on your chart that corresponds to your temperature and day of cycle.

o Many thermometers keep the temperature displayed until you use it again, so you don't have to record it straight away if it is still dark or you are trying not to wake your partner.

o Your temperature needs to be taken ideally at the same time each morning after at least five hours consecutive sleep. Mark your regular waking time then record any variation. When you sleep in, record the temperature and adjust your temperature down by adding a second mark .05 (one box lower) for each ½ hour extra sleep and up .05 (one box higher) for every ½ hour you get up before your usual waking time.

o   Conditions that may affect your temperature may include things like a late night, fever, a cold, mouth breathing while you sleep, sleeping in, broken sleep or alcohol. These may cause abnormally high or low temperatures, so it is important to record them for understanding your temperatures when looking back over time.

o   Where there is no thermal shift, it is likely ovulation has not occurred.

Your practitioner can use the charts to find out other useful information related to your fertility and make recommendations accordingly. For instance, consistently lower temperatures may indicate a problem with metabolism and thyroid function. If a period starts too soon after a thermal shift or if there is an unsteady temperature rise there may be problems with progesterone production which can impact implantation. All these require further investigation before diagnosis, but charting can get us on the right track early when there are issues that may impact your chances of conceiving.

# Sienna's Story

Sienna, aged 38, came to the clinic after trying to conceive for seven months. She had a four-year-old little girl (conceived naturally) and was keen to conceive soon. Sienna had made an appointment with an IVF specialist as she was concerned it was taking a while to fall pregnant, and she was conscious of her age.

Sienna worked in a high-stress sales position and complained of being "more snappy" with her husband and child over the past several months. Due to her high stress she often had a glass of wine to help her relax (6-8 drinks/week). She agreed to stop alcohol and coffee. This had the added benefit of reducing sugar as she took two sugars in her coffee.

After discussing timing of conception, we realised Sienna had some mis-information about her fertile time and had been trying to conceive at the wrong time of the month. They were trying to conceive 10 days before her period, which was after she had ovulated. Her cycle varied from 25-29 days, and after charting her cycle with temperature and mucus we found her fertile window to be between Days 11-15.

Sienna was prescribed some supplements and herbs to support her nervous system and reduce the impact of stress on her fertility. She agreed to start looking after herself more and began with regular monthly massages and listening to the Be Fertile guided relaxation for natural fertility CD most days. After two months she was feeling much more energised and less snappy. She conceived three months after first presenting and interestingly, it was when they were on holiday. Her sub-fertility was likely to have been a combination of things but timing being a key part of the picture, along with high stress and lifestyle factors, especially her alcohol consumption.

# HOW DO I KNOW IF I DID OVULATE?

Ovulation can be confirmed by tracking your basal body temperature and watching for the 'thermal shift' as outlined above.

Medically, the so-called Day 21 progesterone test will confirm ovulation as this is the hormone produced by the ovary after ovulation has occurred. Importantly, this test will only be accurate on Day 21 of a 28 day cycle. The test is most accurate when taken seven days after your egg is released (or seven days before your period) so if you have an earlier or later ovulation, you must know to do the blood test on a different day or it will be inaccurate. For example, if you have a 35 day cycle then you should do the test on Day 28 of your cycle.

# SO HOW OFTEN DO WE DO IT?

Sex three to four times a week or every other day during your fertile window should ensure there will be plenty of sperm ready and waiting up in the fallopian tubes for the release of the egg and the magic of conception to occur. Statistically there is little difference (approximately a four per cent increased chance) in conception rates between daily conception attempts and those who are trying every alternate day. Since many couples may find daily sex increases their stress, sex every other day will be just as likely to get you pregnant.[52] Importantly, the take-home message is to have sex at least every second day during the fertile window.

# IS IT NORMAL FOR SEX TO BECOME A CHORE?

If it is taking you longer to conceive than you expected or you have specific fertility issues that may reduce your chances, even the healthiest relationships can come under strain. Many couples trying for a baby so often tell us they are losing the romance and intimacy from their sex lives. Sex can quickly lose spontaneity and become a mechanical chore.

When Assisted Reproductive Technology (ART) becomes involved, adding financial burden, multiple appointments involving pelvic procedures and the medicalisation of your fertility, the strain is further compounded. These stressors understandably put pressure on your sex life and make for uncomfortable bedfellows. With most forms of ART – IVF included – you don't even need to make love to make a baby, and so many couples find good reason not to bother – too tired, too stressed, too bloated, too painful (physically and emotionally), and sometimes even too scared.

While this is obviously understandable and very commonly reported by couples who are asked about it, difficulty with intimacy and love-making does not contribute positively to making a baby![53] Even with IVF it has been shown that intercourse before a transfer can improve outcomes of a positive viable pregnancy. Incredibly, there are components within the semen that help improve implantation.[54]

## IS THERE ANYTHING WE CAN DO?

Wherever possible, try to be conscious of the effect your fertility focus has on your relationship. If there are negative signs creeping in, do something about it! Spend some time connecting with your partner and enjoying each other away from the pressure of trying for a baby. Pay attention to each other's needs for connection as well as space. Allow yourself some time to relax and let go, have fun together. Don't forget or neglect intimacy with each other outside of the fertile time.

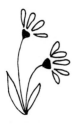

# TIPS ON TAKING THE PRESSURE OFF;
## BRINGING SPONTANEITY BACK.

o   Take time to enjoy each other and the life you have now.

o   Plan for regular date nights or a date weekend.

o   Do fun things! Think about what you used to find fun and rediscover the reasons you got together in the first place.

o   Find ways to make each other laugh.

o   Physically nurture each other with long hugs, massages, take a bath together.

o   Change the time, setting and length of time that you normally make love.

o   If you are finding it all too stressful, then it may be helpful to take a break from charting your cycle for a month or two, still enjoy regular sex three to four times a week.

o   Read our chapter on Stress (Chapter 5) and incorporate some of the suggestions and activities there.

o   Take a break. Couples often tell us that having a break from 'baby-making sex' for a few cycles can also relieve stress by not having to worry about whether they are trying during their fertile time.

All stress-reduction measures can contribute positively to your relationship and your libido. Meditation, exercise, dancing, laughing, yoga, ensuring good quality sleep and time in nature to wind down are all worth considering making more time for. Your fertility naturopath or Chinese medicine practitioner can help support individual factors with specific herbal medicine and nutritional supplements to support the impacts of stress and libido or other health-related concerns that may affect your conception attempts.

When the issues are bigger than the things that you can control, or resentment is starting to build for any reason, it is so important to seek support as early as possible. Find someone that you can (ideally both) talk to comfortably and explore the issues impacting your sex life. Couples or individual psychology or counselling are good first options for support. Group work such as your local IVF support group or women's or men's group can also be a useful resource as discussing your issues with people who will lend an ear, understand and likely even share similar stories can help you feel less alone and more normal.

Infertility is often one of the first real-life stressful situations that a couple has to face together. It can be the breaking point for some relationships but it does often seem to come back down to the impact on intimacy and sex. It certainly deserves important consideration. This challenge can also deepen and strengthen a relationship when faced fully together, with open communication, understanding, support and love.

Life is bound to throw many more difficulties your way, and how you face this as a couple will show you how you will face other challenges in the future – like parenting!

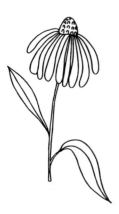

# FAQs from our patients

## Orgasms, sexual positions, lubricants and lying down after sex: separating fact from fiction

### Are any sexual positions better than others for conception?

The number one thing to get right for conception to occur is timing. Any position that works for you where the ejaculated sperm is released into the vagina can lead to conception. Deeper penetration to the cervix is recommended so that the sperm get past the more acidic environment of the vagina. Some experts recommend avoiding positions where the woman is sitting or standing at the time of ejaculation as gravity will draw some sperm down and away from the target. Intercourse can be in whatever position you like, but perhaps at the time of ejaculation it would be a good idea to move to missionary (man on top), side lying or rear entry positions to take gravity out of the equation and give the sperm a swimming chance. This is only a suggestion and in no way a necessity as the sperm are pretty good at swimming in the right direction!

### Should I lie still for a while after sex?

You do not need to lie down after sex to ensure the sperm reaches its destination. Sperm is ejaculated in a viscous substance called semen. The sperm and the semen separate after ejaculation and the sperm swim up through the cervix and into your uterus to start the massive journey to meet your egg! The semen will run out and may have some sperm left in it, but these are not the ones you want so it isn't a problem. A little rest and snuggle after sex is great for your hormones and stress levels so feel free, but it is not necessary for getting sperm to the egg.

## Am I more likely to conceive if I have an orgasm?

The short answer is no. While lacking in evidence, some people believe the orgasmic contractions of the uterus and cervix may help to draw the sperm towards the egg. It is not necessary however, for a woman to orgasm to conceive, but it is obviously a bonus if you can.

## Is it harmful to sperm to use lubricant?

Did you know that most lubricants contain spermicides? This means they can actively damage and destroy the sperm and help to prevent conception. When choosing a lubricant, choose one that is fertility friendly but ideally avoid using them around your fertile time as it will change the pH of your vagina.

# TOP TIPS FOR HER

When you start trying to conceive, try to keep hold of the understanding that you would like to conceive sometime over the course of the year. Remember, you have a 20% chance of conceiving in any one natural cycle.

The best chances of conceiving occur with intercourse within the two days leading up to ovulation or on the day of ovulation – your fertile window.

Day 1 of your cycle is the first day of your menstrual flow (not spotting) and the last day of your cycle is the last day before your next flow. If you regularly have a 28 day cycle, ovulation will generally occur at Day 14, so your optimum fertile window starts at Day 11. This does not apply for cycles that are not regularly this length.

Understanding signs of ovulation, your individual mucus changes and timing your sex to the fertile window will give you an increased sense of confidence in your conscious conception.

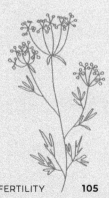

# TOP TIPS FOR HER

Charting your temperatures across cycles provides useful information above and beyond simply knowing your day of ovulation and getting the timing right. An experienced practitioner will be able to determine a range of other potential issues from the pattern of your temperature changes.

If your cycle is different each month or you don't produce fertile mucus or see other menstrual issues, you can obtain good support and treatment from your naturopath or Chinese medicine practitioner. Simple approaches can help with cycle regulation, ovulation induction, fertile mucus production, PMS and other hormonal imbalances, all of which can impact on your fertility.

Try to be conscious of the effect your fertility focus is having on your relationship and your sex life too. If there are negative signs creeping in, don't wait to do something about it.

When the issues are bigger than the things you can control, or resentment is starting to build for any reason, it is so important to seek support as early as possible. When there are difficulties in trying to conceive it can be a pathway to deepen and strengthen a relationship when faced fully together with open communication, understanding, support and love.

CREATE A FERTILE LIFE

# TOP TIPS FOR HIM

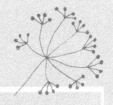

When you start trying to conceive, try to keep hold of the understanding that you would like to conceive sometime over the course of the year. Remember, you have a 20% chance of conceiving in any one natural cycle.

Sex three to four times a week or every other day during your partner's fertile window should ensure there will be plenty of sperm ready and waiting up in the fallopian tubes for the release of the egg.

If you have sperm issues, try ejaculating daily for five to seven days prior to a conception attempt. Research has shown there may be beneficial effects on sperm DNA.

Even if you are doing IVF, intercourse before a transfer can improve outcomes of a positive viable pregnancy as there are components within the semen that help improve implantation.

Talk to you partner to understand when she is ovulating. Getting the timing right is essential for conception to occur and the more you understand about her cycle the better.

If you are having issues with erectile dysfunction or impotence, then please seek professional help from your GP and ask your naturopath or TCM Practitioner for advice.

# 3

# Smokes, booze, and caffeine: the bad guys

When you are at the stage in your life where you are consciously intending to create a baby, you really are ready for life change at many profound levels. While no one can ever really tell you what life is going to be like on the other side of bringing your baby into the world (though they will try) you know that things are going to be quite different from the way they are now.

The moment you make the decision to try to conceive is the moment you need to start making change. "So soon? But the baby isn't even here yet!" The baby hasn't formed, but the start of your baby, the egg and sperm that carry all the genetic data to make your whole baby are maturing in your body up to 100 days prior to the moment of conception. Everything you do in this time affects those two cells — pickle them in salt, trans fats, sugar and alcohol and they are less likely to reach optimal health.

For a woman, once conception has occurred, everything you put in or on your body has the potential to become a part of your baby. For men, until a live baby is squirming in their arms, it can feel hard to relate much to the process. But what happens before conception is integral and both of you need to be on board to make a healthy baby.

When making your baby, you want sweetness and spice and all things nice – there isn't much room for the bad guys here! The changes required to improve the quality of your eggs and sperm affect your health, your healthy pregnancy and birth, the health of your baby into old age and even the health of your baby's children. It is mind boggling to think you can have that much influence over the health of your family for generations to come.

Every day you have the opportunity to make improvements in the choices you make for your diet, lifestyle, general health and, importantly, your fertility. Every day you are faced with a range of options that will challenge your resolve.

We have no doubt some of the suggestions here will feel more like a burden than an opportunity! Some of our patients have no problems making these changes when they understand the benefits or consequences some of their choices have on their chances of conceiving a healthy baby. Some find the changes easier than others. Other people will resist and find it too difficult to make any changes and no amount of research or sensible thinking will help them come around. This is especially true when addiction is involved of course; however, it can also be true for various other social or emotional reasons.

When seen as an opportunity for growth, understanding of your health and empowerment for improving your chances of success, these changes can be much easier to embrace! While you may not have understood the effects some of these things have had on your health and your body in the past, giving yourself the opportunity to really get it now will affect your choices for life. The increased tendency for healthy choices will also mean this level of understanding can be passed on to your children.

# CIGARETTES: "IS SMOKING REALLY THAT BAD FOR MY FERTILITY?"

There is no good news about cigarettes – except the news that another person has quit smoking. We all know that smoking is harmful to us, and hopefully you know that it is harmful to your fertility as well.

Here are the hard facts on smoking and fertility – and they may be difficult to hear!

**Female smokers:**

o   Take longer to conceive.[55]

o   Are twice as likely as non-smokers to be infertile (60% increased risk of infertility).[56]

o   Have an increased risk of miscarriage and ectopic pregnancy (with the risk increasing with each cigarette smoked: there is a one per cent increase in risk per cigarette smoked per day).[57]

o   Are more likely to suffer implantation failure in IVF and poorer embryo quality.[58]

o   During pregnancy are more likely to develop complications such as birth defects, low birth weight, placenta praevia, placental abruption, premature labour and eclampsia (a life-threatening pregnancy condition).[59]

o   Accelerates the loss of reproductive function and may reach menopause one to four years earlier (or for passive smokers, 1 year early), not ideal when you are trying to conceive![57,60]

o   Increase the DNA (genetic) damage in the egg.[57]

> **Interesting fact:** smoking is associated with a thicker zona pellucida (the outer shell of the egg).[61] This is the outer layer that the sperm must penetrate in order to fertilise the egg. Thus, the thicker it is the more difficulty the sperm will have, making it less likely conception will occur. It is the same impacts for active and passive smoking.

## Male smokers are more likely to have;

o   Impotence and erectile dysfunction (not helpful when you are trying to conceive!).[62,63]

o   Poorer sperm health (on all semen parameters including numbers, motility and morphology).[62,64]

o   Increased DNA (genetic) damage in the sperm.[65]

We also know that even if a woman doesn't smoke but her male partner or sperm donor does, she is much less likely to conceive naturally or with IVF, and is more likely to miscarry.[66–68] Passive smoking or exposure to second-hand smoke (work or home) has also been shown to increase the risk of miscarriage, stillbirth, and ectopic pregnancy (i.e. passive smoking is only slightly less harmful than active smoking).[67,69]

## If you do manage to beat the odds and conceive, if either parent is a smoker at the time of conception, it is likely to substantially affect the health and well-being of your baby, with increased risk of:

o   Small babies (and all the associated health complications).[69]

o   Asthma, decreased lung function.[70]

o   Sudden Infant Death Syndrome (SIDS).[71]

- Birth defects (e.g. cleft lip and/or palate).[72]

- Leukaemia and cancer later in life.[66,73]

- An increased risk of neurological and behavioural issues e.g. attention deficit disorders, impulsivity, etc.[74]

- Increased risk of smoking as an adult (double the risk).[75]

- Increased risk of most psychiatric disorders during adulthood.[76]

- For female babies, smoking impacts negatively on the development of their ovaries.[77]

It is good to know that although most of the effects of smoking on your fertility will be reversed one year after quitting, you will experience improvement with every week that goes by without a cigarette. The effects of passive smoking are not much different to actively smoking yourself, so it is a good idea to remove yourself from any smoky environments and encourage your smoking partner to quit. The benefits to fertility start immediately.

## Do I have to give up completely or is the occasional cigarette ok?

To achieve the best impact on your fertility you do need to quit completely.[78] Having the occasional one or two cigarettes often leads to an increase in cravings and stronger withdrawal symptoms and makes it more difficult to quit entirely. Also, the risk of miscarriage and/or ectopic pregnancy increases with every single cigarette you smoke. If you also consider the harmful chemicals entering your body (lead, cyanide, nicotine etc.) and the impact this has in reducing the oxygen supply to the eggs and sperm, then the sooner this exposure is ceased the better.

## I know I have to quit but I'm struggling

Giving up is not easy! It is certainly much easier if you know why you are doing it and you have a goal to achieve – a healthy, happy bubba.

What will support your intention to give up the smokes for good?

## Helpful hints to give up those cigarettes for good

| | |
|---|---|
| **WHEN** | Identify when you are likely to have a cigarette or feel like a cigarette. |
| **WHY** | Consider why you feel like smoking at those times. |
| **HOW** | Think about how you can avoid those scenarios/situations or put in place alternative options. How can you distract yourself from the moment of smoking and then replace smoking with an alternative positive action: glass of water, a walk, anything but a cigarette. |
| **WHAT** | What will you replace it with that provides a sense of purpose and fulfillment to motivate you? What will motivate you to be healthy? Could it be a new hobby or passion? Hanging out with non-smoker friends, exercise, dancing, the thought of making your child... |

For example, if you only tend to smoke when you drink alcohol, then avoiding the alcohol is a good start. Or if you know that you smoke when you are stressed then read through our chapter on Stress (Chapter 5) to come up with some great solutions that should help make it easier. If certain people or situations weaken your willpower, it might be good to avoid them for a while until you get the cravings under control and can easily say no.

We had one patient who realised she only really smoked to escape from work. Having a cigarette break was a way for her to get out of the office and away from a job she hated. Upon this realisation, she began looking for another job and fortunately was lucky to find one she enjoyed relatively quickly. She had stopped smoking for good by the end of the first week at her new job.

However, not everyone will find quitting smoking as easy as finding a new job (and looking for a new job isn't necessarily easy either). If you are struggling to give up, then go to the experts. Good and proven options for support in quitting smoking include:

o   Quit Line (in Australia) call 13 78 48.

o   Acupuncture.

o   Naturopathy.

o   Hypnotherapy.

o   Nutrition.

o   Counselling.

Along with a useful website, Quit Line also has a free app (MyQuitBuddy) you can download that helps support you in your journey towards a smoke-free life.[79] You can program the app so that it sends you alerts during your 'danger times' that remind you of why you need to quit. It also helps you set realistic goals as well as gain support from others. It can be a useful addition to your quit smoking program.

# ALCOHOL: "WHERE'S THE HARM IN A LITTLE DRINK?"

While some couples may consider sharing a bottle of wine as part of the romance for getting in the mood to make a baby, there is now enough evidence from research to suggest that *no alcohol* consumption is the only safe level for women when trying to conceive or when pregnant. Indeed, these are the guidelines recommended by Australia's National Health and Medical Research Council.[80]

Did you know that alcohol consumption can decrease your fertility?

Women who abstain from alcohol (or decrease their alcohol intake) whilst trying to conceive have double the chances of conceiving compared to those who don't alter their drinking habits prior to commencing fertility treatments.[81]

## Effects of alcohol on fertility

### In women, alcohol may: [82-83]

o   Impair ovulation, fertilisation and implantation.

o   Reduce your chances of conceiving.

o   Increase your risk of miscarriage.

Did you know that alcohol affects male fertility as well?

### In men, alcohol may: [84]

o   Reduce testosterone.

o   Reduce sperm production.

o   Contribute to impotence and ejaculation problems.

## Surely an occasional drink is ok?

For the biggest boost to your reproductive systems and your best chances of conceiving a healthy baby, it is ideal if you can avoid drinking at all for at least three to four months while your eggs and sperm are developing leading up to conception. In our experience, those who make the necessary lifestyle changes (which includes abstinence from alcohol) are the ones who usually experience the best success. We recommend that men continue to avoid alcohol until their partner is safely into the second trimester, especially if there has been a history of miscarriage. Alcohol is such a problem for developing babies that ideally women should avoid alcohol until your little one has been weaned from your breast milk to avoid any exposure at all.

## I know I should stop all alcohol but what are the guidelines if I choose to have the occasional drink?

There are some occasions where having a drink feels like part of the celebration. It is all about being selective about which occasions you choose, as it is possible to find a reason to have an alcoholic drink every weekend or even every other day. If you find yourself in circumstances where you would like to have a celebratory drink, restrict your overall intake to no more than two standard drinks per week. Remember, a standard drink is not a full glass!! It is just 375ml of beer, 100ml of wine, or 30ml of spirits. And it doesn't accumulate! If you miss one week, you can still only have two drinks next week.

For the potential mum, if you have already ovulated and are waiting for a pregnancy test result, it is best to avoid it all together. During pregnancy, complete abstinence is recommended.

## HOW MUCH IS A STANDARD DRINK?

| | |
|---|---|
| Can/Stubbie low-strength beer | = 0.8 standard drink |
| Can/Stubbie mid-strength beer | = 1 standard drink |
| Can/Stubbie full-strength beer | = 1.4 standard drinks |
| 100ml wine (13.5% alcohol) | = 1 standard drink |
| 30ml nip spirits | = 1 standard drink |
| Can spirits (approximately 5% alcohol) | = 1.2 to 1.7 standard drinks |
| Can spirits (approximately 7% alcohol) | = 1.6 to 2.4 standard drinks |

## What to drink instead? Water!!

Most alcohol substitutes are full of sugar so best avoided for healthy hormones, weight management and stable blood-sugar. Water is your best option. If you are out at a bar or function, try mineral water for some bubbles and mix with a bit of juice if necessary - pink grapefruit or cranberry juice are often your best options. Put it in a champagne glass if it helps to feel like more of a treat! Avoid mocktails as they mostly always contain sugar syrup, and sometimes some nasty flavour or colour additives too.

Pairing your new non-drinking habits with other new activities is a great way to stay on track. Try to identify the times you are more likely to have alcohol. Is it at the end of a stressful day to help you relax? Or, is it only when you socialise? Identifying the 'danger times' and why these are danger times for you can be instrumental in finding alternatives and solutions to assist in giving up the booze. (The 'when, why, how, what? tips in the smoking section above can help provide you with more useful tools).

Instead of sitting in front of the TV with a beer or going out for dinner and sharing a bottle of wine, you might choose to exercise in the evening and eat a healthy meal or go for a walk together after dinner. You will often need to change your normal routine/pattern. This will support your overall health levels, weight management, and help distract you from any drinking habits you may have.

## Karen's Story

*Karen came to the clinic when she was trying to conceive and although her cycle had always been regular, she had noticed that in the last six months her periods had become irregular. Around six months earlier Karen lost her job and a family member passed away, resulting in Karen becoming depressed. Her diet and lifestyle changed dramatically, she was regularly consuming at least one bottle of wine every night, unhealthy snacks throughout the day and only one main meal. Karen was also a vegetarian but was not eating any vegetarian protein options. She admitted being too tired and sad to cook and that she had a history of using alcohol as a support if she was depressed. Karen had also gained 10kgs in the previous six months, which undoubtedly contributed to her depression.*

*Karen and her naturopath discussed the effects of alcohol and inadequate nutrition on menstrual cycles and hormonal balance in women. She was advised that it wouldn't be an ideal time to conceive at this point and was encouraged to see a psychologist for extra emotional support.*

*Karen's desire to become pregnant motivated her to change and she was able to reduce her alcohol intake. In addition, supplements were prescribed to help support her mood, improve her blood-sugar balance and replenish the nutrients missing from her diet.*

*After several regular visits, Karen's diet had evolved to three main meals (all of which included good sources of protein) and five alcohol-free nights (her alcohol consumption had reduced to two drinks on the weekends). Her periods had resumed their previous 28 day cycle and she was feeling more stable in her mood and herself.*

*From here Karen started trying to conceive again with the goal of stopping alcohol completely. Four months later, Karen had conceived and had been able to maintain her diet and a stable mood.*

---

## COFFEE AND CAFFEINE: THIS TOO?

The safest option is to cut out coffee prior to conceiving. This is not only due to an increase in the chance of miscarrying, but it appears caffeine also delays time to conception. In a scientific review, women drinking over 300mg/day of caffeine (2-3 cups of coffee) had a 27% lower chance of conceiving each cycle and those having less than 300mg had a 10% reduction in conception rates compared with women consuming no caffeine.[85] What this basically means is it may take longer to conceive if you drink coffee.

There is also evidence that women are more likely to miscarry if they regularly consume caffeine in their pregnancy: 200-300mg/day (2-3 cups/day).[52] In one meta-analysis, the authors found that for every 100 mg/day increase in caffeine intake in early pregnancy, the risk of spontaneous abortion increased by 14%.[86]

For men, research shows that drinking more than 2 cups of coffee per day significantly increased the rate of miscarriage in their partners, thought to be due to potential DNA damage to the sperm.[87,88]

A Brazilian study has also linked lower fertilisation rates with ICSI for men doing IVF and drinking coffee. [89]

Regular use of caffeinated products is double edged. As a diuretic, coffee also increases the excretion of water-soluble nutrients such as folic acid, B vitamins, vitamin C and other important nutrients required for optimal reproductive function.[90]

As we want to maximise your fertility we recommend limiting consumption of any caffeine-containing products to an absolute minimum and consider cutting it out altogether whilst you are trying to conceive. This is most important after ovulation – when it is possible conception has occurred – due to the risk of miscarriage.

### Is decaffeinated coffee ok to drink instead?

Whilst choosing decaffeinated coffee is a far better option (ensuring you are having chemical-free water filtered organic decaf), there may still be some drawbacks. It is possible that other compounds in coffee may have less-significant anti-fertility effects, including possibly increasing the acidity of the fertile mucous, compromising the sperms ability to survive in the female reproductive tract.

Some types of decaffeination use nasty chemicals too. Organic, water-filtered decaf coffee is a better option if you are struggling in giving up that morning ritual. Try to keep it very occasional.

### How much caffeine is in my diet?

Caffeine is found in coffee, chocolate, cacao, most energy drinks, black, green and white tea.

| FOOD | CAFFEINE CONTENT[91] |
| --- | --- |
| Espresso | 145 mg/50 mL cup |
| Formulated caffeinated beverages or 'Energy' Drinks | 80 mg/250 mL can |
| Instant coffee (1 teaspoon/cup) | 80 mg/250 mL cup |
| Black tea | 50 mg/250 mL cup |
| Coca Cola | 48.75 mg/375 mL can |
| Milk chocolate | 10 mg/50g bar |

As you can see, it doesn't take much to get up to a higher caffeine level in your diet. E.g. one espresso in the morning, an instant coffee in the afternoon and a bar of chocolate after dinner will mean you have consumed at well over 200mg caffeine for the day.

## Using tomorrow's energy today

We regularly consume caffeine products such as a café latte or some chocolate to boost our energy. It does this by driving our adrenal system to produce more stress hormones, thus giving us an instant boost. Our muscles contract, heart rate increases, our liver releases sugar into the bloodstream and blood flow slows to reproduction and digestion systems as well as skin to maximise flow to the brain and essential organs. If we use this to fight an attacker or flee from a scene, we will find that we fight harder and run faster. But if we are consuming caffeine on a daily basis – especially without the physical energy expulsion – we are more likely to head towards burning out our adrenal system, gaining weight and feeling more tired after a very short-term boost (if anything at all). We call this using tomorrow's energy today, which means that ultimately you can't catch up and may even need to keep increasing your caffeine intake to feel the hit or get satisfaction.

Intuitively we know that stress is not good for fertility and essentially your daily caffeine habit is fuelling an increased stress response in your body. Longer-term effects of drinking coffee include muscle twitching, insomnia, difficulty with digestion, nervous tension, anxiety and even panic attacks with a sense of impending doom. It makes sense, therefore, to break the habit of your daily coffee to assist you in reducing stress and anxiety.

### I want to stop my coffee habit, but I'm worried I won't cope well with withdrawal symptoms

Most people find the first three to five days of caffeine withdrawal the hardest. Headaches are the main symptom that will tempt you to have just one more coffee but if you can persist you will find that you start to feel much better without it. Our patients report with happy surprise that they are less stressed and anxious, more stable, have consistent energy through the day and a better night sleep to follow. All of this will mean a natural increase in energy you could not possibly achieve with coffee and you will be soon convinced that you are better off without it!

Herbal teas are a great substitute. Dandelion Root tea can be a good coffee substitute. It doesn't taste like coffee and is disappointing if you expect it to! But it does have the bitterness of coffee, can get your bowels going (a reason many of our patients say they drink coffee) and you can add a little milk of your choice to make it feel more like a satisfying drink. You probably won't like the first cup much, so start weak and build up. It has a nice nutty, malty, toasty flavour so after a few cups you may find that you start to like it! Most people find they do enjoy it if they persist every day for a week – then it can become your regular hot drink.

Alternatively, there is now a huge range of herbal teas available on the market, shop around and find one you love. An easy one to get hold of is Rooibos tea, a South African herbal tea that is readily available in the supermarket. As a bonus, it has a great range of antioxidants and contains no caffeine.

> Our recommendation for women trying to conceive is no coffee while for men one coffee per day. We suggest limiting caffeine (in all its sources). Stick to no more than one to two cups of weak tea per day and restrict other caffeine such as chocolate to the occasional treat rather than a daily fix.

## MARIJUANA: ARE MY EGGS/SPERM 'STONED' TOO?

This is the most commonly used illicit drug amongst people of reproductive age, and is worth discussing as it is linked to decreased fertility in both men and women and dramatically affects the quality of sperm, and impacts negatively on the health of developing babies during pregnancy.

In men, THC (the active ingredient in marijuana), weakens sexual drive and reduces sperm production by interfering with the production of testosterone. Sperm party hard too – research has shown that they become hyperactive, swimming too hard too early and burning out before they reach the egg.[78] Yes, every cell in your body becomes 'stoned' and if sperm don't have the energy left by the time they reach the egg, they don't have a chance of breaking through the outer casing of the egg for fertilisation to occur.

Women who smoke marijuana also secrete small amounts of THC in their vaginal fluid and reproductive organs, and when the sperm come into contact with it, they go into party mode, becoming hyperactive and burn out too quickly.[92] Marijuana can also harm a developing baby, especially in the first weeks when you may not even know you are pregnant.

## Consequences of smoking marijuana on fertility

### In men:[92,93]

o   Reduces libido and sexual function.

o   Decreases fertility.

o   Reduces the number of sperm produced.

o   Reduces capacity of sperm to fertilise the egg.

### In women:[94–96]

o   Reduces chances of conception.

o   Reduces the numbers of eggs retrieved in IVF.

o   Reduces chances of healthy pregnancy associated with implantation failure, spontaneous miscarriage, foetal growth restriction, low birth weight babies and premature birth.

Of course, some men who smoke marijuana do get women pregnant, but every man has a different fertile potential and it changes throughout his life. If your fertility is already compromised, smoking marijuana will make you infertile. Women who smoke can also conceive, but as for men, if your fertility is already compromised by any factor, or your man's fertility is poor, smoking marijuana will make it very difficult to conceive, reducing your chance of having a healthy baby.

**If you are trying to conceive we recommend that you
don't use marijuana in any form**

Aside from the above risks, marijuana may also be contaminated with problematic heavy metals (such as lead to increase its weight and sale value per gram, which also adversely impact your fertility and health) or more addictive illicit drugs, such as cocaine. It's just not worth it.

Research is tricky to conduct on the singular impacts of marijuana on fertility specifically, as people who smoke or consume it tend to higher rates of cigarette smoking, alcohol, caffeine and other illicit drug use before and during pregnancy. Of course, marijuana is often smoked in combination with tobacco and this has its own inherent fertility disasters too.

# WHAT ABOUT OTHER DRUGS?

Party drugs, street drugs, illicit drugs such as cocaine, speed, ecstasy, heroin and ice all have dramatic effects on fertility and, of course, your overall health. Men may suffer reduced libido, abnormally-shaped sperm and low sperm count. Women often suffer abnormal ovulation and irregular menstrual cycles as well as a reduction in ovarian reserve. Long-term use can lead to permanent problems, but in many cases, any damage caused may start to reverse as soon as you quit your habit.

Results from research may be confusing; however, the growing body of evidence suggests that to produce optimal outcomes for healthy pregnancy and baby, women and men should be encouraged to avoid all forms of substance-use behaviour while trying to conceive (and ideally before) and during pregnancy.

# WHAT ABOUT MEDICATIONS?

If you are taking medication for a health condition, consult your doctor to check if it has any known detrimental effects on fertility – they may be able to offer you an alternative. Some drugs that can affect ovulation in women include: aspirin, steroids such as cortisone and prednisolone, tranquilisers or seizure-prevention medication, thyroid medication at the wrong dose and, of course, any hormonal medication including oestrogen or progesterone (including pills, creams and patches).

Some of the drugs that can affect male fertility include certain high blood pressure medications (such as calcium channel blockers and angiotensin converting enzyme inhibitors), antipsychotics, tricyclic antidepressants, chemotherapeutic agents, anabolic steroids, testosterone, antibiotics, ketoconazole and sulfasalazine. Medication for hair loss can also impact on sperm production. Consult your GP for a medication review and get a second opinion from your pharmacist.

# MY FUTURE BABY

With the regular use of any addictive substance during pregnancy, your baby must suffer the withdrawal symptoms after birth that you are avoiding yourself. After getting your baby used to regular doses of these substances, even though some will cross to the breast milk (compared to being more directly attached to your blood supply) there is a dramatic reduction in exposure. This means your baby suffers severe headaches, pains, shakiness, emotional turmoil – all of this while getting to know the feeling of life on the outside. What a difficult start to life for all of you! There is no better reason to give up now! Giving up now is not more stressful than the potential poor health outcomes you are creating for yourself and your baby.

# WHAT IF I AM ADDICTED? HOW CAN I GIVE UP?

Stay motivated. Get support. Join a group. Be kind to yourself but stay on track. Remind yourself why you are doing it. Reward yourself regularly. Save up the money you don't spend on these things and treat yourself to a massage or even a holiday! Do the maths – most people don't realise how much these habits are costing them! Literally put the money aside and use it to reward yourselves every week or month that you stay on track.

Support for detoxification with naturopathic work can help by improving elimination, reducing suffering experienced during withdrawal while also reducing cravings and dependence. Acupuncture and hypnotherapy have been shown to significantly reduce cravings.

With our patients we often find that emotional reasons underlie substance use. We try to duck and weave away from our feelings and fears by masking them or pushing them down with a cigarette/ a drink/a shopping spree/a food binge... (or insert your special avoidance tactic here).

Counselling can be very useful to identify the ways in which we hide, what in fact we are hiding from and how we can show up to and resolve these issues without the need to dampen it down. You may have tried this in the past and didn't find it worked for you – don't give up! Try someone else, something else to give you the support you need to make the change. You know these things are harmful for you, your fertility and your baby. Now is the time to work on this and it will make the inevitable stresses of early parenting easier too.

> You don't have to wait for a chronic health condition or a diagnosis that frightens you to make these changes – let the thought of creating a baby from your own cells and DNA drive your desire for change. Start now.

## What can I do to help give up my addiction to caffeine/alcohol, etc.?

o Get support from a friend or a support group.

o Follow the **WHEN**, **WHY**, **HOW** and **WHAT** outlined in the above smoking 'helpful hints to give up for good' section.

o Remind yourself why you are giving up.

o Reward yourself regularly.

o Seek counselling.

Take a good look at the reasons you feel you need to consume these things at the time you usually would. Do you feel socially awkward, inhibited or less interesting? Do you feel tense and hard from a busy, stressful week? Do you feel left out of the gang if you don't partake? Are you bored? Do you want to escape a moment or a conversation? What are some other ways of dealing with these feelings?

Many people worry/wonder about how they are going to stay focused on their abstinence in social situations when their friends/peers are doing what they are trying so hard to avoid. In the early days of change it is a good idea to avoid situations that will tempt you and throw you off the wagon. If you are feeling terrible from detoxing/ withdrawing, you will be easily persuaded to have that thing. Just this once... Perhaps lead the way by trying to organise other activities such as going to a day spa or having lunch (rather than dinner) where it is easier to avoid drinking.

If you do need to go along, try to be clear about why you are doing what you are doing before you enter into these situations. If you feel you can't divulge why you are not having a drink or a smoke when you usually would, just tell them you are doing a detox for your health and ask for their support in not offering you another one. Of course, if you feel you can tell them you are trying for a baby, most likely everyone will be supportive and either congratulate you on your choices or ask you for your reasons (in which case you may have the opportunity to educate someone else on the benefits of avoiding these things when they come to trying to conceive!).

Support your partner. If you are both doing this together, you can be each other's rock in these situations – when one of you weakens, the other can be strong.

## I HAVE GIVEN UP ALCOHOL AND COFFEE, BUT MY PARTNER HAS REFUSED. IS IT WORTH IT IF IT IS JUST ME MAKING THE CHANGES?

If your partner, whether male or female seems resistant to making lasting change, remember that one very good quality egg or sperm is better than two dodgy gametes! Ideally, we recommend both partners make changes and the best results definitely happen under these circumstances. Persist in making yourself as healthy as possible knowing you are still making a significant impact on the health of your baby. Your partner may be inspired to make changes when they see how positive the changes are for you. Ultimately, every little bit helps.

If one partner isn't as committed to making these changes as the other, for whatever reason, then this can be a real source of tension in the relationship. Someone who is really making an effort will feel undermined, unsupported and may even begin to question whether the other person is as committed to making a family as they are. They may question whether they are the right person for them to be making a baby with. We see patients in this kind of dilemma all the time. Good counselling support is paramount to either sort out problems such as different priorities, objectives or beliefs or making the decision to move on.

# IT GETS EASIER!

*"By being open with family and friends about what I'm doing, people tend not to tempt me. Also, after such a long time without it, I've gotten used to not drinking, and the desire to do it has dwindled."*

**Isobel**, FGHG patient

It gets easier to live without these things in your life. While it may be hard to imagine when you first start making the changes, most people find they feel much better for it. So often there can be a good snowball effect where positive change gives energy and inspiration for more positive change. We've often had patients tell us how much more energy they have since they have quit (especially alcohol); they usually report a clearer head in the morning, a better libido and stronger focus and concentration during the day. When we are consuming these substances on a regular basis we are not aware of the impact it has on the way we are feeling on a day-to-day basis.

How much will you save? Add it all up and put the money towards positive healthy change. A massage, a holiday, a facial, a personal trainer, regular acupuncture or your nutrients and herbs.

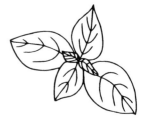

# TOP TIPS FOR HER

Take steps to eliminate addictive substances that are harmful to you, your developing eggs and your baby, particularly cigarettes, alcohol, coffee, and marijuana. Ideally this should be done before your three to four months of preconception care prior to trying to conceive. The longer the better.

Remember the safest levels of these drugs for women is zero whilst trying to conceive, during pregnancy and whilst breastfeeding.

Consult your GP to review any over the counter or prescribed medications you may be taking to ensure they have no known effects on fertility.

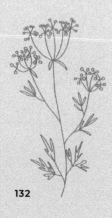

CREATE A FERTILE LIFE

# TOP TIPS FOR HIM

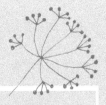

Ideally eliminate alcohol consumption to protect sperm and testosterone production while trying to conceive. Remember to keep consumption to a minimum until your partner is well into second trimester – especially where there is a history of miscarriage.

Eliminate cigarettes and marijuana intake completely.

Limit coffee to one a day or fewer.

Consult your GP to review any over the counter or prescribed medications you may be taking to ensure they have no known effects on fertility.

Consider these changes to be your contribution to supporting your partner. If IVF is part of your journey, she will endure a barrage of tests, invasive procedures, appointments and stress. Your support will make the world of difference to her coping and endurance, help you to conceive more quickly and have fantastic outcomes for your healthy baby! Think of yourself as a father now.

# 4

# Exercising for fertility: your fertile weight

We've all heard the statistics about weight and obesity, and we can all agree they're pretty scary. But are you aware of the impact weight has on your fertility? Are you aware that fertility for both men and women is drastically compromised by being overweight or obese? If you know weight is your issue then our recommended diet chapters (Part 2) and our chapters on blood-sugar, inflammation and hormonal health (Part 3) is essential reading for you.

## FOR WOMEN

There is little doubt that obesity is one of the biggest causes of infertility in Australian women. Overweight women are more likely to take longer to conceive, have hormonal imbalances and irregular ovulation (including insulin resistance and PCOS).[97] The risk of pregnancy complications is also much higher, with overweight and obese mothers more likely to miscarry or suffer stillbirth, high blood pressure, pre-eclampsia, gestational diabetes, blood clots and require higher intervention in labour and birth as a result.[98] Further, children born to overweight mothers are more likely to develop obesity and Type 2 diabetes later in life.

So you can see why we are super keen to talk about reaching a healthy weight wherever possible when trying to conceive.

## Consequences to female fertility
of being overweight or obese [97-98]

- o Increased time to conception.

- o Lower rates of natural conception.

- o Higher risk of miscarriage and stillbirth.

- o Poor IVF outcomes; higher rates of cancelled cycles, lower rates of success.

- o Increased risk of pregnancy complications (high blood pressure, gestational diabetes, blood clots).

- o Poor health outcomes for children (increased risk of obesity, Type 2 diabetes).

## FOR MEN

The impacts of carrying excess weight for male fertility are perhaps less widely discussed; however, they are actually significant, and comparable to those effects for women. Overweight men are more likely to suffer from lower sperm counts, and also poor results in all other semen parameters.[99]

But the major impact appears to be an increase in DNA damage within sperm, caused by what's known as 'reactive oxygen species' (ROS): damaging substances associated with the inflammatory processes of obesity and insulin resistance that cause oxidative damage to cells in the body.[100] This not only leads to increased time that it takes to conceive, but also increases the chance of miscarriage resulting from fertilisation from these sperm.[101] And even more concerning, Australian researchers have recently found that children of overweight fathers are far more likely to suffer from insulin resistance and obesity, as well as reduced fertility in later life, particularly boys.[102]

Recently some interesting research from IVF clinics in Adelaide has shown drastic impacts to IVF outcomes with overweight men. Researchers found that outcomes were poor, even when female partners were of a healthy weight. They also found that embryos created from overweight men were less likely to develop properly and were less likely to lead to a successful pregnancy. This is all due to DNA damage.[101]

Another major issue for overweight men is the impact on hormone levels. High levels of fat lower testosterone and cause an increase in oestrogen production. This hormonal imbalance is associated with poor sperm count, low libido and erectile dysfunction, increased risk of cardiovascular disease, a loss of muscle mass, depression, fatigue and poor vitality.[100] Including a reduced chance of fathering a child, this is a significant multi-symptomatic condition for men, and the benefits of healthy eating and exercise cannot be overestimated in preventing and reversing these issues.

## Consequences to male fertility
## of being overweight or obese [99-102]

..................................................................

- o Low sperm count.

- o Poor quality sperm.

- o Low libido and erectile dysfunction.

- o Increased time to conception.

- o Reduced conception rates.

- o Increased miscarriage rates.

- o Poor IVF outcomes.

- o Poor health outcomes for children.

# WHAT IS A FERTILE WEIGHT?

From a fertility point of view, it is important to know whether you are in a healthy weight range or not. The calculation known as the body mass index (BMI) is often dismissed as inaccurate, but for ninety per cent of us the BMI is a realistic calculation to assess our ideal weight. The types that possibly don't score accurately include muscular people (those who are naturally stocky, or those who do a lot of muscle building exercise) and women who are particularly hour-glass in shape (tend to hold weight at their bust and hips). Otherwise for the rest of us, there isn't really a reason to discredit this calculation. The healthy weight range is a BMI from 18.5-25 and this is the ideal range for healthy fertility too.

# Sonia's Story

*Sonia, age 36, presented with severe obesity (BMI of 35), PCOS, and low energy. She consulted us for help to improve her health and her chances of conception prior to a frozen embryo transfer. Sonia had a 3-year-old daughter and 20-month-old son both conceived via IVF and had one frozen embryo remaining. However, after an unsuccessful frozen embryo transfer three months earlier, her periods had not returned.*

*To help improve Sonia's hormonal balance and encourage the return of her cycles, she was prescribed herbal and nutritional medicine alongside dietary and lifestyle changes. In addition, she had regular acupuncture with one of our colleagues at FGHG. Sonia was highly motivated and lost two kilograms in the first two weeks by increasing her dietary protein, reducing her carbohydrates and exercising four to five times a week. Within the first month she had lost 7.5kg and reported a significant improvement in her energy levels. Her periods returned in the second month of treatment and she continued to lose weight.*

*Sonia then prepared to have her remaining embryo transferred; however, despite thawing successfully, the embryo was found to have abnormal cells and thus was not able to be transferred. Consequently, the resulting disappointment led to a 5kg increase in Sonia's weight. After her next appointment with us, she became even more determined and as they were now preparing for a fresh IVF cycle, focus on improving her husband's sperm health was also recommended. He also followed a specific program including herbs and supplements, and an increased exercise routine.*

*Three months later, Sonia had lost the additional 5kg she had recently gained and had decided to start trying to conceive naturally whilst waiting to start another IVF cycle. Happily, they didn't get to that next cycle as they conceived naturally in that first month.*

*They went on to have a beautiful, healthy baby girl, and are still awestruck that they fell pregnant on their own after so many years of IVF.*

---

# EXPLAINING THE BODY MASS INDEX (BMI)

As mentioned earlier in the book, BMI is calculated with this formula: weight (in kilograms) divided by height (in metres) squared. For example, a 75kg woman who is 156cm tall, has a BMI of 30.86 (75kg/1.56x1.56 = 30.86) and is considered obese. For her height, her suggested healthy weight range would be between 45-60.6kg

There are a range of very convenient BMI calculators on the Internet – just make sure you know your height and weight before you look one up!

---

**BMI RANGES**

**< 18.5**: underweight | **18.5 – 25**: healthy weight
**25 – 30**: overweight | **30-35**: obese | **> 35** morbidly obese

---

It has been shown that women who experience ovulatory problems due to insulin resistance can significantly boost their fertility by losing 5-10% of their body mass. For example, if you weigh 80 kilograms, that would be four to eight kilograms of weight loss. For many women, this is a far more achievable goal than working towards an ideal body mass index prior to conception. One recent study that looked at overweight women found that those who lost 10% of their body weight had significantly higher rates of conception (88% versus 54%) leading the researchers to suggest that all health-care providers should incorporate weight loss counselling when treating overweight patients trying to conceive.[98]

Just as with female fertility, it appears that men also experience some of the benefits of weight loss by losing 5-10% of their total body weight.[97] It is likely that many of the issues associated with obesity are related to insulin resistance, and this destructive blood-sugar pattern will start to improve on the day you make positive changes to your diet and lifestyle.[102] What great news! You have some control over your outcomes!

When it comes to IVF, there is now a lot of convincing research to suggest that BMI significantly affects outcomes. One large 2012 American study found that overweight women were between 37% and 68% less likely than healthy weight patients to achieve IVF success, depending on their BMI. The higher their weight, the less chance they had of achieving pregnancy.[97]

Research also shows a significant increase in the incidence of miscarriage associated with increased BMI. Every point above a BMI of 25 increases the risk of pregnancy loss.[103]

It is important to note that there are concerns around weight loss and potential damage to egg or sperm quality. Rapid or recent weight loss may damage maturing eggs that are being prepared to be released or developing sperm. In an ideal world, it is better to lose weight, and then wait for another three or four months to allow your egg and/or sperm quality to recover before trying to conceive. This will further reduce your chance of miscarriage. However, if time is of the essence (i.e. age is a significant factor) gradual weight loss with good liver and antioxidant support from your naturopath is the safest option.

# HOW TO LOSE THOSE EXCESS KILOS!

So it's all well and good giving you lots of depressing statistics on the impacts of excess weight, but what about the nitty gritty of how to lose those pesky or seemingly stubborn extra kilograms? We see a lot of men and women who have been struggling for a long time with their weight. Generally, they feel as if they've lost control, and may have tried many types of complex diets but haven't had much lasting success. At the end of the day, there is no special trick, formula or pill that is going to work when it comes to weight loss. Whilst there are some medical problems that can impact your ability to lose weight (e.g. hormonal imbalance, thyroid problems etc.) it all comes down to the basic 'calories in, calories out': how much you eat and how much you move!

But we can give you some specific tips and insights that you may not have been aware of until now.

Generally, to achieve weight loss, you need to follow a healthy diet combined with regular exercise. For more specific tips and advice about how to lose weight safely, please read the "how much exercise do I need to do?" over on the next page, and also read on to the diet section outlined in Part 2 on the fertility diet.

# BUT ACTUALLY, I'M SKINNY!

The 'Fat is Fertile' motto belongs to times gone by when food was less available, and our lifestyles were far more active. Many women were underweight and to be 'fat' was probably actually being in the healthy weight range with a few more curves than just skin and bones.

Being underweight reduces your chances of conceiving a healthy baby, as irregular or absent cycles are a common effect of a low BMI.

To remain fertile it is thought that women need to carry a minimum of 22% body fat.[104] We have all heard the stories of female athletes losing their menstrual cycles as they train hard, but it is also possible for those of us who are just mere mortals and go a bit too hard with exercise, lose too much weight or are already underweight and have ovulatory or luteal phase issues. You may even experience fairly regular menstrual cycles, and not be aware that you are not ovulating.

As fat cells contribute to our oestrogen supply, some fat is essential for achieving adequate oestrogen levels to achieve ovulation. Without enough oestrogen, your ovaries will not be stimulated for a fertile cycle and will not release an egg. Your body simply does not have the resources available to maintain a regular healthy ovulation and menstruation cycle. As a consequence, women with a BMI of less than 18.5 are twice as likely to take more than a year to conceive compared with healthy-weight women.[105]

Research has shown that low-fat diets may also contribute to ovulatory disorders. For example, studies have now shown that by eating low-fat dairy foods you may be doubling your risk of infertility.[106] Good fats, are part of a well-balanced diet, and essential for achieving adequate hormone production required to achieve regular ovulation, and therefore enhance your chances of conception.

## HOW MUCH EXERCISE DO I NEED TO DO?

When it comes to exercise, there are many differing opinions on how much and what types are best for you. The answer, more often than not, is that most people are not doing enough exercise. We always encourage our patients to look at their exercise levels in terms of what we were built to do. Our physiological requirements for health have barely changed in the past few thousand years, but our lifestyles have. Dramatically so in fact. We were not built to sit on our bums all day, with only the occasional attempt at physical activity. We were built to move: to walk, to run, to squat, to lift, to climb, to jump. And we were built to do this for a fair chunk of the 16 hours a day we are awake.

For the best health and fertility benefits, it is important to engage in both cardio and weight-bearing exercise. Cardio is the sort of exercise that gets you sweating and your heart pumping. Running, fast walking, cross trainer, rowing, swimming, aerobics, netball, tennis and dancing are all classified as cardio exercise. Weight-bearing exercise is the type that challenges your muscles and increases your strength, including yoga, pilates, weight lifting and body-weight exercises.

## GUIDELINE TO EXERCISE REQUIREMENTS TO IMPROVE FERTILITY

| MY BMI (MEN AND WOMEN) | GENERAL GUIDELINES |
|---|---|
| 18.5-25 | You are in the healthy weight range, so your goals are to maintain this and to help improve blood flow to the reproductive organs on a regular basis. Aim for >30 mins x 5/week. |
| > 25 | You are in the overweight/obese range and need to lose weight to help improve your chances of conceiving. Aim for 60 mins per day or four sessions of high intensity interval training (20-30 mins) per week. |
| < 18.5 | You are underweight and need to increase your body weight to help improve your chances of conceiving. Avoid high intensity exercise and instead focus on gentle exercise only e.g. walking, gentle yoga etc. |
| I'm male | In addition to following the relevant guidelines above, you also need to avoid any exercises that will compromise sperm health i.e. cycling (the pressure and increased heat in the testicles is associated with sperm damage and decreased fertility). |

CREATE A FERTILE LIFE

The recently updated Australian Government health guidelines recommend physical activity every day, and around two and a half to five hours a week of moderate intensity activity or one and a half to two and a half hours of vigorous intensity physical activity or a combination of both — and so do we.[107] This does not mean you have to go to the gym for one hour five days a week but you do need to get moving. The type of exercise and the frequency will also depend upon whether you need to lose weight or not. If you are a non-exerciser, you may start with something like the seven-minute workout (an app you can download and do anywhere, anytime), which gets your heart rate up and gets you moving initially for just seven minutes at a time.[107] Other times it may be an hour of walking, or three separate lots of 20 minutes throughout the day. Research has shown that meaningful weight loss, and improvements in fertility, can occur with just 30 minutes of exercise five times a week (150 minutes a week).[98] Refer to the above table or your health practitioner for specific guidelines that are appropriate for you.

As we've said, your exercise will need to depend on your fitness level and general health. An example for some of you might look like this. A daily 30-45-minute brisk walk or cycle to work and a 15-minute walk in the park at lunchtime. Then ramp up the cardio and weight bearing exercise for around 45 minutes three times a week — this may be an exercise class, yoga, swimming, dancing, running, gym, tennis or a team sport. On those days your incidental exercise or a walk to the park at lunchtime will make up your hour.

We need to add a note of caution here. More exercise is not better. If we over exercise this, too, can reduce our fertility. So regular movement and exercise in moderation is what you're aiming for.

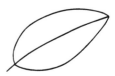

# WHERE DO I START?

o Increase incidental exercise (see below).

o Schedule exercise into your weekly routine.

o Commit to a type of exercise you can continue long-term.

o Work out what's going to motivate you e.g. a dance class, salsa, belly-dancing or Bollywood.

o Find a friend/family member to exercise with e.g. go for walk together (a lovely way to have a social catch-up instead of meeting for coffee).

o If you need extra support, seek help from a professional for an individualised routine e.g. personal trainer or exercise physiologist.

# HOW TO INCREASE INCIDENTAL EXERCISE

Recent research has shown that even getting up from your desk and walking around the office for a couple of minutes every hour can benefit your blood-sugar and triglyceride levels.[108,109] So have a think about what you can do through the day to increase your incidental exercise:

o Move around the office.

o Don't book the meeting room: if meeting with just one or two others, go for a walk instead of sitting down.

o Walk around when you're on the phone.

o Take a break for a drink of water.

o Use the stairs.

o Walk to the train or the shops.

o Ride instead of drive to work.

- Park your car a few streets away from your destination.

- Walk around the block in your breaks.

- Walk to the park or a cafe farther away in your lunch break.

- Stretch your body between tasks.

- Stand wherever possible.

- Sit on a fit ball instead of a chair.

- Buy a pedometer, a fitness wrist band or use an app on your phone to motivate yourself to get up to 8,000-10,000 steps a day.

- Download an app that reminds you to get up and move regularly.

- Challenge yourself to undertake incidental exercise at least five times per day.

# I'M STRUGGLING TO ACHIEVE THE NECESSARY AMOUNT OF EXERCISE

You are not alone! It can be really difficult to balance work, family, life and exercise. It can be useful to write a list of the reasons you think explain your lack of exercise. Gradually work through each option as if trying to resolve it on behalf of someone else. Work through your list and find solutions to all the excuses. If you really don't know how or where to start, enlist professional help. A personal trainer, a coach or even a fit friend can be a great start.

Regular exercise is not about motivation, it's about discipline and routine. It's the same thing that ensures you clean your house, go to work, wake up in the morning and have a shower. Sit down with your diary and mark in the times during the week you will do exercise, just as you would a meeting or an important project. And then just do it. Don't think about it. Don't build dread before you even start by thinking it over. Don't bargain with yourself or start thinking you should prioritise other things. Just go.

Recognise it may be a challenging hour, but also understand it is only one hour out of your entire day, and when it's over, you're finished for the day, and you can feel great about yourself as you go on with other things! Remind yourself of the benefits rather than the detractions and remember that the more you exercise the easier it gets to exercise – fit, healthy bodies like movement and activity, in fact, they even crave it!

This really is your opportunity to give something incredible back to yourself. To amaze yourself. To be proud of your success. Because you can do this! Every one of us – no matter our apparent limitations – can do this in a way that works for us. And despite the fact you think you may hate exercise, once you become a fitter, happier, healthier person, you will learn we all have great capacity to love physical activity, or at least its benefits. And really, what else in your life can you do for only a few hours a week and obtain major results? It's actually the most efficient investment you can make! If only building a career and creating/managing a family were so easy!

# AND ANOTHER BONUS

Do you know all the benefits of exercise?

## Exercise

....................................................................................................

o   Improves mood and sense of well-being.

o   Improves bone density.

o   Slows the aging process.

o   Improves sleep.

o   Reduces cholesterol.

o   Improves libido.

o   Improves blood sugar control.

# HOW CAN EXERCISE
# IMPROVE MY FERTILITY?

Most importantly, when it comes to starting a family, men and women who exercise are benefiting their fertility in a number of very important ways. By improving blood-glucose regulation and assisting in healthy weight maintenance, exercise assists in regulating ovulation in women and improving sperm health in men. The research convincingly shows that couples who exercise have increased fertility and conceive more quickly, and better health outcomes for both pregnancy and their children.[45,98]

By building stamina and strength three to four months before you conceive it will help achieve a good pre-pregnancy weight and you are more likely to keep active and fit during your pregnancy. This is great preparation for the birth and then carrying your baby and coping with everyday life. Building abdominal and lower back strength is also likely to reduce the risk of you experiencing lower back pain during pregnancy. And of course, all of this bodes well for birth and caring for a newborn.

So what's not to love? Imagine how healthy and fit you can feel, not to mention the benefits of improving your chances of conceiving.

Remember we're not talking about training for a marathon, a 100km walk or Iron Man here. Not even a six-day-a-week boot camp. Those would be detrimental to your fertility.

## Benefits of fitness/exercise on fertility

- Ovulation regulation.
- Reduced miscarriage rates.
- Enhanced sperm health.

- Enhanced libido.
- Quicker time to conception.
- Reduced risk of developing diabetes and hypertension in pregnancy.
- Improved birth outcomes.
- Improved health outcomes for children.

# A NOTE ON EXERCISE AND IVF

How much exercise should women be doing when they are trying to conceive, especially when they may be pregnant or after an IVF transfer? This is difficult to give advice around because every individual is different.

# RECOMMENDATIONS FOR EXERCISE DURING IVF

As a basic rule, if you are already an exerciser, you can continue to exercise after you may have conceived or after your IVF transfer, but at a reduced rate.

Moderate your exercise depending on your symptoms and fitness levels.

**After egg collection:** gentle exercise ONLY for a few days after egg collection, no matter how well you feel.

**After embryo transfer:** ONLY gentle walking for that day and walking a few days after.

**Thereafter:** moderate, gentle exercise is fine, but be conscious of overheating, heart-rate and over-exertion.

It is very important to be conscious of your temperature, as overheating is associated with pregnancy loss. We suggest you don't exercise so that you feel hot, sweaty and breathless — a good rule of thumb is to make sure you can still talk when exercising. It is also important to exercise to the point that you feel well and energized afterwards, rather than exhausted and avoid exercising outside on a very hot day. If you are used to measuring your heart-rate during exercise, aim to keep it at about 80% of what you can usually comfortably do. Earlier guidelines recommended keeping heart rate below 140 beats per minute; however, current guidelines suggest moderate-intensity exercise rather than focusing on heart rate.

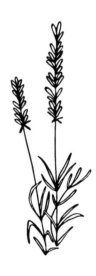

# TOP TIPS FOR HIM AND HER

If you are overweight, reducing body weight by as little
as five per cent can significantly improve fertility
and pregnancy outcomes.

If possible, drop weight before trying to conceive or wait
three months after significant weight loss to resume trying.
If time is of the essence (i.e. age is a significant factor)
gradual weight loss with good liver and antioxidant support
from your naturopath is the safest option.

If you are underweight, consider reducing your exercise
intensity, and review your healthy food intake, especially
healthy fats. Improving your stress management and
sleep may be helpful too.

Aim for regular exercise incorporating planned exercise
activity and incidental exercise. The frequency and type will
be dependent upon your current body weight and health.

Don't wait for motivation to strike.
JUST DO IT! Prioritise and diarise.

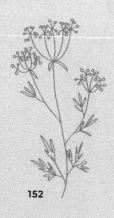

CREATE A FERTILE LIFE

# 5

# Befriending stress to enhance your fertility

I f you have been trying to conceive for a while - no doubt you have heard it all:

*"Just relax and it will happen!"*

*"I had a friend who was trying with IVF for five years before giving up and then they conceived – accidentally!"*

*"I heard about a couple who were trying to conceive for years, doing everything right. When they went on holidays to Bali, they let it all go and got pregnant!"*

Maybe you have even heard of the IVF clinic that has set up in the Caribbean to take advantage of these sentiments? While relaxation and stress management are an essential part of preparing to conceive, it can often add to the stress and frustration to hear comments like this and becomes yet another way we can be hard on ourselves.

While well-meaning friends and family are often feeling impotent themselves in finding a way to help you, these kinds of clumsy comments grate at the edges of most people who are doing all they can to have a baby.

Stress is a normal part of our life, it is a motivator, helping to enhance our performance — both physically and mentally — and helps us meet deadlines. Although the reality is, in our everyday life we can lurch from one task to the next creating a busy world for ourselves — and a busy mind. It is such an everyday part of life that learning about the impacts of stress can feel scary, especially when you are trying to conceive, and don't know what to do about it.

**Is the high level of stress in your life playing a part in your fertility problems or do the fertility problems create the additional stress?** Both of these may be true and certainly the longer you've been trying the more likely you are to have stress as a contributing factor in failing to conceive. Stress causes a hormonal cascade to help us cope by directing energy and circulation to our brain and muscles and away from non-essential organs like the reproductive system. This affects the regulation of our hormones, blood-sugar and adrenal function, and it's well established that our reproduction is compromised, especially when experienced long term. In our more stressful months we might have a 40% reduction in our chances of conception if we're stressed during our fertile window.[110] It makes sense to address our stress for our overall wellbeing. When researchers suggest that women who wish to conceive may increase their chances of getting pregnant by taking steps towards addressing stress like exercising, talking to a health professional or engaging in a stress-reduction practice, then it makes sense to start today. [110]

**Remember to be gentle on yourself while you read this.** Trying to conceive can be one of the most stressful times, especially if it is taking longer than you ever imagined, but there is hope! Maybe it is time to reframe how we relate to and think about stress.

# HOW DO I KNOW MY LEVEL OF STRESS?

Many of us know the tell-tale signs of stress when under pressure but others are so used to feeling that way that their high-stress lifestyle feels normal. Which is it for you? Have you experienced any of the following 'significant life stressors' in the past year?

o Marriage or divorce?

o Moved house?

o Death or illness of a friend or family member?

o Lost your job?

Or other stressors such as:

o Serious deadlines at work or with study.

o Financial worries.

o Emotional stresses from family and relationships.

o Being ill.

Major life events are one sure way to know your body is likely to be under more stress than normal, and for many, just trying to conceive is a major life event. Answering yes to any of the above scenarios means you have been dealing with what are considered 'major stressors' and thus higher levels of stress.

However, apart from the major stressful situations, we are all under constant physiological stress in the world we live in. We are affected by light, sounds, traffic, pollution, television and the technology we use, always checking our phone or emails and now, social media seems to take up every spare space in the day. This assault on our senses ensures we constantly live with a heavy baseline of physical and mental stress and then any emotional turmoil adds an additional layer. Then there is the extra load we may put on ourselves: training for a triathlon, doing punishing workouts at the gym, burning the candle at both ends to fit in social occasions or the latest binge watch TV series (just one more!), too little sleep or being constantly busy and eating nutritionally-poor foods!

Even if things are generally feeling relatively easy right now, with no major life issues going on, take a look and see the modern-day activities that may be having an impact. Go back to the questionnaire on stress at the start of the book to double check if stress might be hampering your chances of conceiving. It's a growing need for us all to learn to create opportunities to redress this balance whenever we can.

# WHAT IS THIS THING CALLED STRESS?

It is important to know that the body doesn't differentiate between physical stress such as marathon running, long working hours, a traumatic life event or even a past event that you worry about and mull over and over in your mind. Our 'fight or flight' response is a physiological reaction in response to a perceived threat to our very survival. This response can be activated by many events including our feelings of being overwhelmed, irritated, frustrated, anxious or constantly ruminating about negative thoughts. In this fight or flight state, we may feel tense or alert (to fight off the threat or flee from the scene), and our sympathetic nervous system will send out acute impulses to pump stress hormones like adrenaline and noradrenaline into our bloodstream which cause an increase in heart rate and blood pressure, sweating, and muscle tensing. We might have intense focus (causing difficulty sleeping and zapping energy) or trouble focusing on unrelated small tasks. At the same time, our 'non-essential' organs like digestion and reproduction are slowed as they are not important for survival in an acute threat situation. It is important to see how the physical chemistry for our bodies is the same no matter what the trigger.

# HOW DOES STRESS
# IMPACT YOUR FERTILITY?

## Betty's Story

*Betty was a lovely 32 year old, a gentle and kind-hearted woman. She was very slim and petite, and had been diagnosed with PCOS. She had an irregular cycle that was significantly affected by stress. Her cycle ranged from 35 days through to around six months. She had been trying to conceive for two years without luck.*

*She embarked on herbal treatment and acupuncture and managed to regulate her menstrual cycle resulting in a 35-40 day cycle with regular ovulation. After a few months with no pregnancy, a fertility specialist recommended Betty take Clomid (clomiphene citrate) for three cycles to stimulate ovulation. Still no pregnancy, and the specialist recommended IVF, which Betty didn't feel ready for.*

*Stress was mounting at work and around her fertile window when they were trying to conceive, so we discussed the possibility of taking some time off work to relax and calmly focus on becoming pregnant. Betty chose to leave her stressful job, and the change was dramatic. Within two months her cycle was consistently under 30 days, and the following month she became pregnant.*

Unfortunately, we grossly underestimate the impact stress has on our menstrual cycle and our ability to fall pregnant. Of course, we are not suggesting we all go and quit our jobs but taking the time to address stress is crucial. This may mean taking up a regular yoga class, meditating, gardening, walking... whatever soothes your soul.

In the busyness of life, often juggling home and work pressures, we can spend more and more time in the 'fight or flight' mode of being. Under stress, the innate intelligence of the mind and body directs the focus of physiology towards other aspects of keeping our bodies working (i.e. to heart and muscles as described above), so the reproductive function gets pushed low down on the priority list. There is less blood flow and therefore oxygen and essential nutrients to reproductive organs.

## Stress can be associated with

**For women**

o   Less than optimal development of the endometrium (the lining of the uterus), follicles and eggs.

o   Missed periods or irregular periods.[111,112]

o   Reduction in conception.[110,111,113]

o   Damage to egg quality with increased stress hormones like cortisol depleting oestrogen.[114]

o   Poor egg maturation, reducing fertilisation and pregnancy rates[114]

**For men**

o   Less than optimal spermatogenesis and compromised sperm production. Some research has shown that the stress from fertility treatment and IVF can negatively impact sperm quality.[116]

**For Both**

o   Poor lifestyle choices, which in turn affect our reproductive physiology and add to the risk factors for conception and pregnancy.[115]

o   Poor long term health outcomes for the offspring.[116]

Stress triggers a cascade of events resulting in the adrenal glands becoming overworked and, potentially exhausted over time. The initial adrenalin rush is one we all recognise and occurs to alert us to imminent danger. This is useful when we need to perform, such as a work presentation or reacting to an emergency to provide energy, strength and focus, but it should be short lived. When stress becomes chronic, it results in continually elevated adrenalin and cortisol. These hormones raid our stores of nutrients leaving us feeling wired and/ or exhausted and may lead to frustrating symptoms such as poor sleep, weight gain and poor immune function. These elevated stress hormones result in less of the building blocks needed for oestrogen and progesterone, which are crucial hormones of fertility. So our busy life is potentially robbing us of a healthy balance of reproductive hormones.

In addition, the effects of acute or chronic stress on sex drive and libido is something many people report. Obviously, that is the last thing you need when trying to conceive!

## GOOD NEWS: EMERGING SCIENCE IS STARTING TO SHOW US A NEW WAY OF THINKING ABOUT STRESS.

Recently, scientific research has shown that stress is most harmful to us if we believe it to be so. This can really help any of us when going through a time of acute stress. While we have long been told that stress is our enemy and that we should just relax, some research now suggests that we can benefit from re-framing it in a more positive way.

Based on her research, health psychologist Kelly McGonigal advocates that we benefit from embracing stress.[117] Instead of being concerned with the levels of stress we are under, she suggests we find a way to change our minds about stress and its effect on us. In real life stressful situations, when we experience sweaty palms and a pounding heart, McGonigal encourages us to think about how these signs show our body is preparing to meet the challenge. It is also very useful to observe how the body's response under pressure can look and feel similar to its response to joy and courage. We can view it as a positive – that we're energised and ready for the situation.

The research showed that when our heart was pounding under the usual stress response, our blood vessels constrict in an unhealthy way. Amazingly, when our heart pounds and we view this as helpful, our blood vessel stays relaxed! It seems the negative physiological changes in our body may happen because of worried thoughts about the stress and whether we accept stress as helpful or reject stress as a poison.

McGonigal goes further to explain that one effect of stress is to encourage us to be more social by the release of the hormone oxytocin (often called the cuddle hormone). This hormone supports us to be more compassionate and caring, and encourages us to seek support from others. More human connection stimulates further release of oxytocin. In times of stress this hormone is pumped out alongside adrenalin. Why? Oxytocin is anti-inflammatory, actually protecting us and our cardiovascular system from the effects of stress. Clever, isn't it? In fact, it can even repair damage to and strengthen our heart – fascinating that a hormone released under stress can do the opposite of what we previously thought! So it seems the stress response has a built-in mechanism for stress resilience. Isn't it great to know that by reaching out to others, we recover from stress faster!

It gets even more interesting, as there are other researchers out there finding that the more connected we are with others, the more we look each other in the eye, the more we touch each other, and the more we help others, the more likely we are to be happy. So this intervention of connection is a super effective way for us to be happier and to deal with day-to-day or bigger life stressors. Reaching out to others, caring for others such as being there for a friend in a time of struggle also releases oxytocin in the body and has the same protective health effects. How lovely that caring for others creates resilience to stress.

## A SIMPLE WAY TO CHANGE THE IMPACT OF STRESS ON YOUR BODY

When you next find yourself in a stressful situation at work or in day-to-day life and you have acute signs of stress (or during any high-intensity moment), the best thing you can do is reframe stress as your ally. Remember, your body is trying to connect to your compassionate heart.

o   Recognise those stress symptoms of a pounding heart or sweaty palms as signs your body is doing a fantastic job of rising to the current challenge. Be thankful to your body for handling the stress.

o   Put your hands over your heart to help evoke a softening and a feeling of kindness to yourself.

Over time, you can learn to trust yourself to handle whatever stress comes your way. Use these powerful tools to negate the negative effects of stress on your mind and body as well as your fertility.

## SUPPORT CAN REALLY HELP

For many people the very act of trying to conceive, especially if finding it more difficult or taking longer than expected, is a source of major stress in their lives. It can also feel very private and many people find themselves isolated and silenced by a feeling they can't share their struggles with anyone – either through feelings of shame, fear of judgement or that nobody really understands. Reaching out to a trusted friend or finding a support group – even online – can be a great way to alleviate the stress and isolation and discover that not only are you in good company but others have the same struggles as you. This can be wonderful for putting things in perspective and reducing your stress levels. If you are having trouble conceiving, you are far from the only one – remember, one in six couples have difficulty conceiving.

## SWITCH ON YOUR RELAXATION RESPONSE AND SWITCH ON YOUR FERTILE POTENTIAL

The good news is that the science developing now is telling us not only that stress is good for us (if we perceive it as such), but also the neuropsychologists are showing us we can use simple techniques to change our mind and our brains. Even in the busiest day, if we can find a moment to appreciate something (anything!) and just stop for 10 seconds to absorb those feelings, it strengthens the mind and gives space for our body to soften. If you can practice stopping for moments like this every day, over time your brain and nervous system will start to rewire, and you will feel more able to cope with challenges that arise during your day.

Alice Domar is a Health Psychologist who has done a series of studies on the impact of psychological interventions on pregnancy rates.[118] Participants doing 10-sessions of mind-body cognitive behaviour stress reduction had a 42% spontaneous conception rate compared to only 11-20% of women in the support and control groups. These were women who had been trying to conceive for one to two years. She has had similar results on groups of women undergoing IVF with pregnancy rates more than double for the mind-body groups.

The mind-body connection can be a key to some people unlocking their fertility. Instead of feeling drained by the antics of our mind, positive neuroplasticity can retrain the way we react and behave. By switching on the 'relaxation response' and switching off the 'fight or flight' response we are allowing the body to be more receptive to conception. Pregnancy is a state of relaxation when the message from the brain is saying everything is 'safe' in our world. The body's innate intelligence perceives physical or emotional stress or worrying as an unsafe time for pregnancy.

By inclining the mind towards expansion, softness, and relaxation and using any of the suggestions in this chapter to get out of the fear zone and into a more relaxed and connected mind and body state you are preparing your body for pregnancy. By choosing a relaxation technique such as guided relaxation you are 'putting your foot on the brake pedal' of your over-activated nervous system and you're using positive neuroplasticity to literally change the way you think — strengthening good habits and new neural pathways. You are being proactive in reducing a heightened nervous system response, which allows your body to function optimally and restore well-being. Switching on the relaxation response on a daily basis is like taking a short holiday every day.

## Give attention to positive moments

We will often spend many minutes reliving stressful conversations or events we wish we could change. If we could spend even a fraction of this time on absorbing and reliving positive moments we would be changing the neural structures in our brain. This alters the brain's natural negativity bias and leaves us feeling safer, more connected with others, and more happy and confident.

- Start to notice moments in your day where you feel good, it may be playing with your dog, noticing blossom on a tree, smiling at a neighbour, birdsong, being praised by a colleague or a friend making you a cup of tea.
- Take a moment to enrich this experience by feeling the experience in your body with all your senses, acknowledging it and letting the experience nourish you. You can do this for 10-20 seconds at the

time of the event, relive the moment later that day or recall one or two of these moments before you go to sleep. The more you draw on all your senses to remember and imagine the colours, smells and feeling in your body, the more this practice will benefit you.

According to psychologist and author Dr Rick Hanson, taking in the good is a simple exercise which helps us to look for small pleasurable experiences, replacing what can be a constant, hypervigilant mind on the lookout for potential threats.

# 15 ways to prevent and relieve stress

The remainder of this chapter is like a shopping list of activities. See what appeals to you and start to introduce one of these mind-body techniques on a daily basis. Start today! We're not suggesting you do them all and in fact if you get bored with one, then switch to something else. There are lots of options and here are some of our favourites:

## 1. MEDITATE FOR 5 MINUTES EACH DAY

Taking time for yourself every day and allowing your mind and body to settle and relax is a hugely positive thing you can do for yourself. The benefits are cumulative and if you take that time to do a relaxation or to meditate you will notice a difference. Even your family and friends may notice a calmer, more relaxed you. You may feel more able to cope with stressful situations, feel happier and less overwhelmed by problems.

CREATE A FERTILE LIFE

# How do I do mindfulness meditation?

**Read and record the following passage on your phone. Remember to speak slowly and ensure there are no loud background sounds. Sit quietly or lie down, take a deep breath and replay your recording.**

1. "Take a deeper breath as you sit up taller, lengthening your spine, with your arms at your sides or gently resting on your belly... Allow your eyes to soften and find a gentle focus... Notice how you feel... Notice how your body feels right here... right now... Are you holding tension anywhere?

2. "Now take a deeper breath in... and as you gently sigh the breath out, relax any tension... Notice it takes no energy to breathe out, simply let it go... Take another deeper breath in and as you sigh the breath out, relax a little more...

3. "Take your attention to any part of the body where you are holding tension and with each exhale you will release a little more... and relax a little more. Feel a wave of relaxation all through your body and let go into the feeling.

4. "Take a moment to notice how you feel right now... just check in... and allow yourself to let go of any concerns you may have about the past or the future... For the next few minutes you are simply going to be present and feel into the sensations of your body... Notice where your body is touching any surface – the chair or the floor... just become aware of the areas of contact your body makes.

5. "Now let the breath settle to find its natural rhythm... Simply notice where you feel the breath in the body... as you breathe in... and out. Simply noticing... If your mind wanders just bring it back to the present moment... and to your breath as you breathe in and out...

6. "If your mind gets distracted by thoughts, simply return your attention to the breath.

7. "As you breathe into the abdomen, take your attention deep within to your womb and ovaries/ reproductive organs... It's almost as if you can feel the oxygen flowing freely there and relaxing more and more with each exhale. Stay with this gentle breathing for a few more minutes.

8. "Now gently move your body, stretch your arms up, rotate your shoulders, stretch your mouth wide and take a yawn if it comes to you... And carry this sense of calm into the rest of your day. Try to be aware what you give this more relaxed state up for and remember how relaxed you can be."

## Guided relaxation tracks and apps can be a fantastic tool

Many people find it difficult to sit in silence and meditate. If that's you then it's easy to download guided relaxations from the Internet, buy a CD or a phone app. Two of the authors of this book have created some specific CDs and guided relaxation/visualisation tracks to support women and men trying to conceive or going through IVF, written specifically for each stage of your cycle and where you are at right now. Go to *www.befertile.com.au* for more information and to download the guided relaxations. They continue into pregnancy and breastfeeding support, and are great assistance for sleeplessness.

**MYTH: To benefit I must do at least 20 minutes of meditation daily**

This is a myth. Even if you do a 'mini meditation' and take a minute a few times a day you can benefit by reducing your nervous-system response. It can be refreshing to know that taking this small amount of time to tune in to your body can have benefits. Before a meal, on the tram, while riding in the lift, at the traffic lights, before a meeting or even taking a moment on the loo!

Notice the way it makes you feel right after you've done it. You may notice a quietness, a settling down. You've just given your over-used nervous system a break. Try it regularly for yourself. There's no excuse – we all have one or two minutes to spare. So tune in to the sounds around you and simply listen for a minute without judgment. If your mind wanders just come back to the sounds around you. Or try meditating on your breath. Simply bring your attention to your breath and follow it for a minute, notice the pathway from your nostrils to your lungs, your abdomen rising and falling. Simple!

# 2. BREATHE FOR FERTILITY

A stressful breathing pattern looks and feels like shallow breathing from the upper chest only, often pulling in the abdomen and raising the shoulders with the in breath. This is a shallow stress breath and is only going to increase the tension in the neck and shoulders and encourage the fight or flight mechanism. Change your breathing by breathing down into your abdomen allowing your belly to fill and your ribs to move out slightly. You will notice a marked reduction in feeling overwhelmed or stressed.

## Finding your breath – a personal reflection

*"One of the most profound things I have ever been taught is how to breathe. Weird, I know, but I had reached my late 20s and had moved up the career ladder but had been unable to manage my thoughts and my mind. I had started to wake suddenly in the night with a strange panic and feeling of not being able to get my breath. I had no idea this phenomenon was quite common and had a name. When I realised I was having panic attacks, I decided to go along to a yoga class to see if that would help. The teacher taught me deep yoga breathing instead of constantly shallow breathing. This was the start of a long love affair with yoga, and as I started to breath in a healthier way I started to panic less and enjoy life more."*

**Gina Fox**, author

Your breath takes oxygen around your body to your vital organs including the reproductive area, carrying rich nutrients for healthy functioning. Along with this physiological aspect to breathe it can also be a gauge of how we feel. Consequently, we can use breath techniques to regulate our very emotions. When we feel as if we are being led by our emotions and reacting quickly or inappropriately, using our breath can create space and calmness. In a study titled 'Respiratory Feedback in the Generation of Emotion', scientists confirmed what yogis and hippies have been saying for years - they found an association between breathing and various emotional states.[119] This research showed that it's possible to change our mood and how we feel by how we breathe.

# How to take a deep yogic breath

- Sit with an erect spine or stand upright so you can breathe fully. Place your hands on the lower abdomen and as you breathe in through your nose, allow the abdomen to rise and the ribs to expand and finally allow the breath to reach the upper chest. Hold briefly before you gently and slowly breathe out, first out of the upper chest, then the ribs and then finally exhale from your lower abdomen. Hold briefly before breathing in again.

- Try counting the breaths if it helps: Take three to four deep breaths, breathe in for a count of four, hold for two and breathe out slightly longer for a count of six, hold for a count of two. Repeat. And repeat again.

- This yoga breathing increases energy, promotes sleep, relaxes the nervous system and helps you feel calm as well as helping to cleanse the body. Hold the in breath for a couple of seconds to let the oxygen send energy to every cell in your body. Hold the out breath for a couple of seconds to encourage a deeper relaxation and release. Be attentive to releasing any tension as you breathe, especially during the holds.

## When should I do this breathing?

Take three to five consciously deep breaths in bed at night, especially if you have problems sleeping. Do this again on waking to give a good start to the day, and throughout the day as you remember. After a week of doing this, you may to notice a difference in your feelings of well-being.

> Other breathing techniques to explore (or Google™): Buteyko, pranayama, alternate nostril breathing (nadi shodhana), breath counting, box breaths, bellows breath (bhastrika).

# 3. TURN OFF THE TECHNOLOGY — BE SMART, SWITCH OFF YOUR SMART PHONE

In other sections of this book we have already spoken about technology as a stress on us physically and mentally. Make a commitment to turn off the Wi-Fi at home after 9pm (or earlier!) to give you a break and help you prepare for sleep. Be sure to keep your phone at least one metre away from your bed and switch your phone off or switch it to flight mode at night – your alarm will still work in the morning. Even better leave your phone switched off in another room so that you're not tempted to look. Make a pact with yourself not to look at your phone or social media as soon as you wake – it can all wait! Try exercising or meditating before you turn it on. Turn off your social media and email notifications so your phone and computer are less distracting and demanding of your time and presence. Have (at least) one day a week where you choose not to turn on your computer or look at emails on your phone. Look for opportunities to leave your phone behind at home or in the car.

## 4. STRESS BUSTING FOODS AND DRINKS

Did you know that a high-sugar and low protein-diet can create a poor emotional response and trigger the stress response? Research suggests that depression may be linked to our diet, and making health changes has a therapeutic impact.[119] In our affluent world there's a tendency to overeat but still be undernourished. That's what a highly-processed, high-sugar diet can do. A lot of fast foods are high in sugar (which stress out our nervous system and messes with our blood-sugar control), high in transfats and high in calories but low in nutrients. However well we think we eat, we can all make improvements. There's a lot of misinformation out there and mixed messages regarding a good diet but reducing processed foods is an easy, sensible approach.

Skipping meals and super low-calorie diets are off the agenda while you are trying to conceive. These diets are highly stressful. Instead, get advice from a naturopath or trained nutritionist to discuss what a healthy, emotionally-stabilising diet might look like for you.

Nourish yourself daily with nervous-system nourishing foods such as oats, yogurt, kefir, nuts and seeds, berries, oily fish, colourful vegetables and calming herbal teas. Follow our suggestions in the fertility diet (outlined in Chapter 9), which includes plenty of good-mood foods and you'll notice a positive effect on your mind and body and especially your overworked adrenal glands and nervous system.

**Kefir (pronounced like ke-FEER) comes from the Turkish word 'keif'**, which literally translates as 'good feeling'. Research shows that in fact it is really good for people who suffer with anxiety – it is both relaxing to the nervous system and improves sleep.[120] A recent animal study has shown potential for anxiety and depression associated with nicotine withdrawal too.[121]

As a protein and nutrient rich probiotic source, kefir helps to balance the microbiome, healing gut issues like irritable bowel syndrome, improving digestion, regulating immune function, allergic response and inflammation. It's also been shown to help balance blood-sugar and reduce sugar cravings.[122] If your anxiety is linked to your gut, inflammation or pain, or peaks when your blood-sugar is low (ie worse when you are hungry or mid-afternoon) then regular kefir consumption may help.

To really slow down from the busy busy world, try making your own kefir. You can buy the grains in the health food store and find a recipe online.

Other fermented foods such as yogurt, miso, sauerkraut, kimchi or tempeh will have good effects too as a healthy microbiome is emerging as one of the most important things you can attend to for a healthy mind – and the different strains will help support the healthiest microbiome. Variety is key.

# 5. DON'T ALLOW YOUR FERTILITY TO BECOME YOUR WHOLE LIFE

If you are finding that the whole of your life is being taken over by your quest to conceive a child then this might be a useful strategy for you. Take a moment to think of the complexity of your life and the different aspects to your day. There's work, your relationship, your family, health and fitness, friends, hobbies or interests, community, social engagements etc. Your plans to conceive are just one part of that and if this is taking over your every waking thought then it might be time to compartmentalise it and give it say 10-15% of your attention. When you find yourself thinking constantly about your fertility, consciously arrest your thoughts and give your attention to something different – preferably something preoccupying that you enjoy doing.

Still go to your appointments and do what you need to do but then leave the fertility issues behind and get passion back into other important areas of your life. Don't put everything on hold. Get on with life, take up that creative hobby or book that holiday. Remember what used to make you happy and do that again!

Giving ourselves the time to get creative can be a mindfulness exercise in itself. By channelling your energy for creating a baby into your creativity, it can give you a sense of satisfaction you may not have been feeling for a while. It can take our mind off other things we're worrying about and allow us a route to freedom, showing us how to enjoy ourselves again. Allow yourself the time to develop a new skill or take up a past creative talent and see what satisfaction can be gained by expressing creativity in a different way.

# 6. CHANGE YOUR BODY LANGUAGE

Our body language has a big effect on how we respond to others, to life situations and also to how we feel. There's emerging research on this to show that our physiology and hormonal balance is affected by how we hold ourselves.[123] So, broaden across your chest, take some deep life-giving breaths, drop your shoulders and put them back, standing up tall but relaxed. Better still, do some star jumps and smile! Your stress hormone cortisol will go down and happy hormones up. What do you have to lose?

---

### How to make your body smile

Without actually smiling, just very slightly engage your smile muscles by deepening the creases of your mouth. You don't need to pull up into a big smile, just sit with those muscles slightly tensioned. Notice how you feel?

This ancient Buddhist practice is a great simple meditation for shifting your energy when you feel inexplicably down. Do it for a few minutes or try to maintain it for your entire lunch break and just notice what a difference it makes to how you feel.

---

# 7. DO WHAT MAKES YOU FEEL GOOD

Whether it's listening to music, dancing, or having a massage, think about what makes you feel happy.

If you love music and dancing put a dance track on every day and let the energy of the music flow through you while you dance for five minutes or more. It's a great stress reducer! If you've always wanted to go to dance classes now is a great time, especially anything that moves your lower abdomen and pelvis - get into salsa, Bollywood or belly-dancing. This gives you a double benefit of reducing stress (the music, the physical exercise plus the social aspect), increasing your sense of well-being and also improving your fertility by encouraging a good flow of oxygenated blood to your reproductive area and all parts of your body.

> Did you know that belly-dancing may have begun as a fertility ritual? Apart from learning sexy moves to seduce your lover, moving the abdomen and hips increases blood flow to the reproductive organs and can increase your libido and desire too.

For others, having a massage gives a sense of relaxation and well-being we don't often feel. It has physiological tension releasing effects and will reduce stress hormones such as cortisol and adrenalin, increase oxytocin and endorphins and improve immunity and circulation. Book in with a good practitioner who practices gentle relaxation, Swedish massage or deep tissue if you prefer or ask your partner to give you a lovely back rub! You could try committing to massage each other's feet with moisturiser and a drop of essential oil before going to sleep every night. There may be other treatments you prefer to help you relax such as acupuncture, osteopathy, Bowen therapy or reflexology.

# 8. TRY YOGA

Yoga is a wonderful stress management and mindfulness practice and research has even proven its beneficial effects on fertility, improving success if ART or IVF is required and healthier pregnancy outcomes too.[124] Choose your yoga class with your treatment aims in mind. At this stage of your life a gentle, relaxing and calming practice is what is required. Search out a style that embodies a relaxing element and one that works for you. Some yoga centres offer fertility yoga, a more specific style to support your reproductive function. If it isn't available or right for you, consider Hatha, Gita, Yin or Moon yoga that all emphasise these calming qualities. Once you're pregnant it's advisable to find a qualified and experienced pregnancy yoga teacher so you know the practice is going to be suitable for the changes you are experiencing. Ideally, find an ante-natal pregnancy yoga class to join.

## 9. EXERCISE FOR FERTILITY

Exercise reduces our stress levels. Do some daily but keep in mind moderation and refer to our chapter on exercise (Chapter 4) for ideas and appropriate levels for you. Moderate exercise moderates stress but too much and your adrenal glands become over used. If you experience post-exercise fatigue rather than enjoying a lift in your mood and energy, then you need to pull back. Exercise will release tension, interrupt your worrying thoughts, lift your mood and reduce stress hormones. If you are not into the habit of exercising regularly, then start with a brisk daily walk and gradually build up to 30-45 minutes a day. You can also increase your incidental exercise by walking to the shops rather than driving, take the stairs, and walk to the park to eat lunch.

If you exercise in the sunshine then you get a double hit to improve your mood. We also know that getting out in nature has a calming effect on our nervous system so walking or jogging to your local park or forest would make the ideal combination.

## 10. NOURISH YOURSELF DAILY

Do something every day just for you. It may just be five minutes or an hour yoga class but make time to nourish you. You are worth it and your mood and others around you will also benefit. Ask yourself what it is you'd like to do today. Would you enjoy a steaming cup of tea in the garden or in your favourite cafe, or read a chapter of your book, listen to music, call a friend or take a long hot bath? Get back to nature. Even a simple act like standing or sitting in the garden or a local park for five to ten minutes, listening to the birds and looking at the trees or flowers and being enveloped in the green-ness of it all is calming on a deep level. Ask yourself every morning – "what can I do to nourish myself today?"

## 11. LAUGH AND BE PLAYFUL!

Have a good laugh and your major stress hormones like cortisol and norepinephrine will lower and you can reverse your stress response. How long will it take? Well according to one piece of research a funny one-hour video will do the trick.[125] The reverse is also true – watching a war film causes mental stress and reduces blood flow so give intense emotional or thriller/action movies a miss.

There is also a small research study showing a link with improving fertility, especially implantation rates, when women see something funny or laugh around the time of an IVF embryo transfer.[126] Probably one of the reasons is that circulation increases, and muscle tension reduces with laughter – all helpful in the fertility story. Certainly, it helps to combat stress. Find opportunities to cultivate your playful side and seek out fun and laughter whenever you can.

## 12. WRITE IT ALL DOWN

Some research by social psychologist James Pennebaker found that if a traumatic event or worrying episode is going around in your mind and you can't let it go then write about it for three to four days in a row.[127] It was found those people's health improved – they visited doctors half as much, their focus and memory improved, they were less caught up in thoughts and were more socially engaged in the weeks following. Try it but don't do it for any longer as it seems that journaling can also make you more focused on the issues rather than letting them go.

> **Journaling for Positive Change**
>
> At the end of the day write down three new positive things that happened today.
>
> Write a short journal about one of the things — replaying positive events in your mind is good for changing the neuroplasticity of your brain towards a more positive outlook.

# 13. STREAM OF CONSCIOUSNESS WRITING

Another way of journaling is to get out of your own way entirely. Use your breath practice to get you in the mood, and have a pen and paper handy. Try not to try to write anything. Let the pen move in your hand and see what is has to say to you. This may seem a little crazy at first, but it can be incredible to see what wisdom emerges from yourself. If you get stuck, simply scribble away until the next stream of consciousness comes on through. It can even be interesting to see what can be made out of the scribble when you look at it afterwards.

# 14. PRACTICE RANDOM ACTS OF KINDNESS DAILY

Praise someone today or make a wish for someone you know to be happy. Helping others to feel good about themselves has a positive effect on us too. It also helps to take the focus off ourselves and our own worries. What else could you do to help make someone's day today? Practicing small random acts of kindness can really lift the spirits of not just the person who is treated to the surprise, but surprisingly to yourself too.

# 15. BE KIND TO YOURSELF

Above all be kind to yourself and use warm, kind tones and language with yourself. There is a huge movement and body of research on self-compassion led by Dr. Kristin Neff (*www.self-compassion.org*). There are 8-week courses in self compassion which have been shown to be a helpful motivator and stress reliever for us in all areas of life. The theory is based on mindfulness and the central Buddhist teachings around compassion.

To start with, begin to act towards yourself as you would towards a dear friend going through a difficult time. Instead of using critical or judgmental language recognise that this is a tough time and using a gentle gesture to yourself like putting your hand on your heart or hugging yourself. This very gesture creates a softening and a lowering of stress hormones.

The next step is to realise that you're not the only person suffering like this and that these feelings are shared human experiences.

The third step is to be mindful of your thoughts and how you're feeling so that feelings aren't suppressed. Accept how you feel and observe and be mindful of not getting caught up in the story and the negative reactivity.

Self-compassion can give us an inner strength to cope with life's difficult times. Take the first move to show yourself more compassion, create a new habit and see how you feel after doing this for a few weeks.

# WHEN WOULD IT HELP TO SEEK PROFESSIONAL SUPPORT?

*"I feel so depressed when I hear of yet another friend or family member who's pregnant or just had a child. I'm happy for them but I don't want to see them or socialise with them or anyone else for that matter".* If this sounds like you then it's time to seek professional help with a fertility counsellor or psychologist as depression will compromise your fertility, your relationship and your life in general.

Other indicators that stress is impacting on your mental health is when your relationship with your partner, friends or family is affected. If you have feelings of despair, envy, hopelessness or often feel sad or unable to find joy in life then you are in pain. Now is the time to reach out for help. Talk to your partner, friends and people on your health team about how you feel. If you don't already have a counsellor or psychologist on your team, it may be time for a referral to help you cope and recover some perspective.

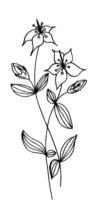

# TOP TIPS FOR HER

Connect with others as a way to reduce stress.

When you're aware of any stress symptoms such as pounding heart or sweaty palms, acknowledge these signs as your body doing a fantastic job of rising to the current challenge.

Counteract your busyness with some deep breaths and make time for meditation or guided relaxations to switch off your stress hormones – even if only temporarily.

Consider downloading a guided relaxation or meditation you can plug in to in a spare moment, before bed or on waking before the day starts and commit to doing it every day. Even if you drive to work, switch off the car then listen to it for 15 minutes before going in to work, you'll find you function better and manage your stress much more effectively.

Quit sugar and highly-processed foods. Instead, nourish yourself daily with nervous-system nourishing foods such as oats, kefir, yogurt, nuts and seeds, berries, oily fish, colourful vegetables and calming herbal teas.

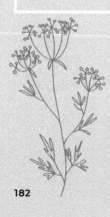

CREATE A FERTILE LIFE

# TOP TIPS FOR HER

Compartmentalise. That is, don't let your fertility concerns take over everything. Engage with it when you need to and then make an effort to be engaged with the other important or enjoyable aspects of your life.

Don't forget to laugh – especially around and after ovulation! Go to see a comedy performance or just hire a funny movie and let yourself enjoy.

Try forming some new positive and stress relieving habits. Read through our list of suggestions, see what resonates with you and start something today.

Read the tips for him – they apply to you too!

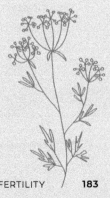

# TOP TIPS FOR HIM

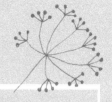

When you get involved in making change to support your conception efforts, you help to ameliorate your partner's stress levels. Your involvement can significantly reduce your partner's stress and will also help you to feel more in control in the process.

Remember your stress levels count too.

When you're aware of any stress symptoms such as pounding heart or sweaty palms acknowledge these signs as your body doing a fantastic job of rising to the current challenge.

It doesn't take a lot of time to reduce your stress and positively affect your stress hormones. Even one minute of deep breathing practiced a couple of times a day will start to chip away at your stress levels. Do what you can.

Reduce stress-promoting foods such as caffeine, alcohol, junk and processed foods, high-sugar foods including soft drinks, cakes and pastries.

Try something different for stress busting and do it with your partner for double the impact. Dancing together is a great way to relieve stress, so consider taking a class. Even just walking together in the evening after dinner is a great method for reducing stress (and waistlines!).

Read the tips for her - they apply to you too!

# 6

# Sleep well
# for your fertility

---

## Martine's Story

Martine had been trying to conceive for six months. She reported a history of anxiety, mood swings (worse pre-menstrually) and lately a depressed mood. Martine used to be a shift worker five years ago and since then her sleep was always interrupted, never satisfying and she could rarely fall asleep before midnight. She now worked in a managerial role that involved a lot of stress.

Martine's diet consisted of quick, easy food that was usually takeaway and although she was home by 7pm, her dinners were usually late in the evening – around 9pm. Often Martine would take her iPad to bed and use the Internet until she fell asleep.

*We introduced Martine to the concept of sleep hygiene, which included eating earlier in the evening, having a strict 'no electronics rule' in her bedroom after 9pm, and we encouraged more 'calm time' before bed. This also involved getting ready for bed 30 mins before her normal bed time and rituals such as chamomile tea, reading a book, doing quick meditations or giving herself a facial or foot massage before getting into bed. She was also provided with some herbal medicine to help support the normal sleep-wake cycle and to help the body cope with stress. Martine began to improve her diet slowly with home-cooked meals where possible with a large focus on getting magnesium and calcium-rich foods into her diet.*

*Martine took on many of the suggestions and returned two weeks later with improvement in her sleep. She could now fall asleep without a problem earlier in the evening and was sleeping through the night 80% of the time. Although Martine reported she found it difficult to not have electronics in her room at night, the benefits outweighed the negatives and she could see it was an unhelpful habit that needed her attention for lasting change.*

*After three weeks more, she reported feeling much more stable with her mood, her anxiety had reduced, and she was waking with plenty of energy in the morning. Martine also had her first period since the changes in her lifestyle and diet and reported that the period was less painful. She experienced a marked decrease in PMS mood swings.*

---

Martine is just one of the many women we see in whom poor sleep is a contributing factor for their fertility issues.

## HOW EXACTLY DOES SLEEP AFFECT FERTILITY?

Actually, sleep is essential for all aspects of health – consider how you feel after just one night of disrupted sleep.

Lack of sleep is essentially a hormone disrupter and will impact on many aspects of metabolism and menstruation.[128] Poor sleep affects the hormone leptin, which in turn affects ovulation and can disrupt all your reproductive hormones, your menstrual cycle, and so also impact your fertility.[129,130] During sleep our body is busily repairing cellular health, detoxifying substances and regulating our hormones. It is essential for optimal fertility for both women and men to get enough sleep.

**Consequences of inadequate sleep on fertility:**

o   Reduces libido.

o   Reduces sexual function (arousal is much more difficult to find when tired or exhausted).

o   Affects ovulation and hormonal balance.

o   Reduces energy and thus reduces likelihood of sticking with your optimal fertility diet and lifestyle choices (we are more likely to reach for caffeine, sweet food or other stimulants after a poor night's sleep).

o   Other health consequences include: fatigue, headaches, weight gain, reduced immune function and resistance to disease, reduced capacity to cope with stress, increased anxiety, reduced lifespan, poor memory, productivity, problem solving ability and creativity.

If you have been experiencing fertility difficulties, then of course stress levels can mount and this in turn can affect sleep patterns. It's common that people trying to conceive – even from their very first cycle – come in to our clinic reporting poor sleep, waking in the night with a stream of constant worrying thoughts. This poor sleep can then exacerbate anxiety and low mood and affect our quality of life quite profoundly. You may need to take some simple steps to manage your stress (see more on this in Chapter 5) and certainly consider if you need more support.

## AM I SLEEPING ENOUGH FOR MY FERTILITY?

Research into a good night's sleep shows that under six hours of sleep is insufficient for most people and over ten hours can also be unhelpful for our mood and wellness.[131,132] For most of us, between seven and nine hours is ideal. Any less than this and your health is being affected.

## HOW MUCH IS ENOUGH?

### < 7 HOURS SLEEP/NIGHT

You are not getting enough sleep, which may adversely impact your fertility as well as your overall health. You need to work out why you are unable to sleep more and take measures to improve your sleep (keep on reading for useful tips).

### 7-9 HOURS SLEEP/NIGHT

Congratulations! This is an ideal amount of sleep, as long as it is quality sleep you are having (meaning you sleep deeply and wake feeling refreshed and relaxed and not tired, clumsy and slow).

### > 9 HOURS SLEEP/NIGHT

You are getting too much sleep, which can also adversely affect mood and overall health. Consult with a health professional to work out if there is a health issue affecting excessive sleeping.

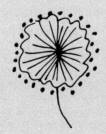

CREATE A FERTILE LIFE

# I DON'T THINK MY SLEEP IS THAT BAD. DO I HAVE A SLEEP ISSUE?

Apart from the number of hours sleep you have each night, there are other factors that suggest you may have a sleep issue. Are you regularly:

o   Getting less than seven or more than nine hours a night?

o   Waking frequently?

o   Taking longer than 15 minutes to get to sleep?

o   Having difficulty getting back to sleep if you wake?

o   Snoring or mouth breathing?

o   Taking medication or herbal remedies for sleep?

o   Waking early?

o   Wake feeling unrefreshed?

Any one of these is a sign you need to take steps to improve your sleep. We know we are getting enough sleep when we can wake naturally without an alarm clock. However, if you wake feeling wired and anxious at 4 or 5am, that is more likely to be a sign your stress hormone cortisol is overworked and you need to de-stress.

It can be the most frustrating thing trying to get to sleep, just lying there tossing and turning all night. There are a number of different types of problems around sleep and some of these can be short lived like being stimulated by a particular incident that happened during the day or something on your mind. The body clock can get disrupted in some cases where you don't feel sleepy at night and stay up late only to find you're unable to get up in the morning. Other sleep disturbances may be things to discuss with your doctor or health professional. For example, sleep apnoea may respond to lifestyle and diet changes, Buteyko breathing techniques or to a device to assist breathing. Depression or anxiety can affect sleep and counselling and other interventions can be needed. If you have pain or experience regular snoring, seek help so that your sleeping can be improved.

A small percentage of the population may have what's called primary insomnia, where they can be high-functioning on only five hours a night but it may still be affecting aspects of health and making some of the changes recommended below may still assist.

## CAN'T SLEEP THEN TIRED ALL DAY?
## IT MAY BE TIME TO RESET YOUR BODY CLOCK

While it is a natural and everyday part of life, many people suffer terribly with their sleep. Many times, we have worked with people in the clinic complaining of insomnia and it is very often simple lifestyle measures that make a difference. If you are struggling with sleep, the first thing to check is your caffeine intake.

If you are sleeping badly, drinking coffee or other caffeinated beverages or so-called 'energy drinks' only makes matters worse. As you are likely trying to conceive, we recommend avoiding coffee and caffeinated soft drinks (please see Chapter 3 for more information) and this is even more important if you are experiencing sleep issues. Although it is preferable to avoid all caffeine (including black tea and chocolate) if you have a sleep issue, don't consume these after lunchtime (drink filtered water or herbal teas instead) and stick to a maximum of two black teas a day.

It will really help if you can become aware of your natural body clock and waves of sleepiness in the evening. Try and ride the wave, listen to your body and go to bed when you feel sleepy rather than falling asleep on the couch or pushing through and then heading off to bed at a later time. A regular sleep routine can work wonders for reprogramming your body clock.

# FIVE STEPS TO RESET YOUR BIO-RHYTHM

In this day and age of electronic gadgets, devices, ubiquitous bright lighting, busy work and social lives, our bodies can lose connection with their natural clock – known as circadian rhythms. Resetting your body clock can be done relatively easily by following this simple exercise for three consecutive days. This is going to be easier to do in the spring, summer or autumn months.

1. **Eat an early dinner** – at least prior to nightfall.

2. **Put yourself in a position where you can see the sun setting.** You don't need to be outside or even watch the entire sunset. Just sit quietly for a few minutes and observe the changing light as day becomes night. This is an ideal time to practice mindfulness – just being in the moment.

3. **Once it is dark, go to bed in a room that is as dark as possible.** Absolute darkness is an important hormone regulator during sleep and any light can interrupt this natural process (some research suggests it can worsen pre-menstrual symptoms and even affect ovulation).[133] Set your alarm for sunrise the following morning (make sure you know what time the sun rises before you go to bed!). Don't worry about the time or the fact that it might be quite early when you go to bed – it doesn't matter if you don't go to sleep straight away. Don't turn on any lights, check your phone, watch TV or otherwise allow yourself to be stimulated. Just lie in bed resting or even meditating or going through your favourite relaxation techniques until you fall asleep. If you are really struggling, listen to a guided relaxation or visualisation to distract you and focus in on deep breathing techniques and switching off. Most people are more tired than they realise, and without constant stimulation will actually fall asleep more easily than they expect.

4. **When your sunrise alarm goes off, be sure to get up straight away.** Don't be tempted to snooze on. Open the curtains or go outside so you can see the sun rising. Again, you don't need to watch the whole thing, though it is a lovely way to start the day. Take 10-15 minutes to be mindful and observe the changing light and sounds as the whole world wakes up around you. This process of observing the changing light is something we evolved doing – electronic light is a relatively new phenomena (historically speaking) and it has drastically interrupted our hormonal and other physiological cues.

5. **Follow this process for three days in a row.** After this time, you should find you are more aware of your end-of-day tiredness, more able to respond to your sleepiness signals, able to fall asleep more easily when you go to bed, and also to wake more easily, feeling more refreshed. You can repeat this any time you find yourself feeling stressed or when your sleep rhythms go awry.

**It is also a helpful practice to reset your body clock after returning from travel – coupled with long walks outdoors in the sunshine, this is one of the best cures for jet lag.**

## WHAT ABOUT A SIESTA?

Luckily research has found that a power-nap during the day doesn't affect our normal circadian rhythm.[134] 10 to 20 minutes will boost energy and keep you alert and you will wake refreshed. A nap for 30 minutes or longer will be restorative but you may wake up feeling groggy. A quick 10-20-minute reset can help decrease stress, let the brain process information and improve productivity, so enjoy it if you have time for a rest. However, don't be tempted to have regular longer sleeps in the afternoon or evening as this can really disrupt sleep.

# How to get the healthiest zzzzzs...

## THE BASICS OF GOOD SLEEP:

### A peaceful bedroom

- It's good to remember that your bedroom is for sleeping and sex! So remove stimulating electronic devices like TVs and computers.

- Encourage relaxation with soft lighting. Lamps or even fairy lights can be nice.

- Make the bedroom a technology-free zone especially no charging your mobile phone by the bed. There's nothing that can't wait till morning so be brave and have a technology clear out. If you are using it for your alarm, get a battery-operated alarm clock instead, or switch your phone to flight mode (although it is still preferable to have your mobile phone out of the bedroom or completely off).

- Is it dark? Heavy curtains, an eye mask or just a piece of soft cloth over your eyes can help.

- Is it quiet? If not try ear plugs.

- Is it clear of clutter and tidy? Creating a safe and lovely bedroom sanctuary that you enjoy being in can help you feel more relaxed and want to get to bed earlier.

### A comfortable bed

- Is your mattress comfortable? Is it time for a new one?

- Is your pillow a good one for you, contoured to your neck and comfortable? Pillows should be replaced at least every three to five years and all bedding should be washed and aired regularly.

o   Is the temperature right for sleep? You may need a summer and winter doona, so you don't overheat or get cold during the night.

o   We spend a third of our lives in bed, and the quality of this third significantly affects the quality of the other two thirds! Worth a little investment don't you think?

## A bed-time ritual

o   Wind down 45 minutes before bed. During this time turn off the TV, mobile phones and computers.

o   Reflect on your day. Think of three things for which you were grateful.

o   Perhaps have a quiet read or even meditate.

o   A cup of quality herbal tea can aid the wind-down. Something like chamomile and lemon balm. Drink it throughout the day or earlier in the evening so you are not woken by your bladder all night!

o   Get ready for the next day. This might include preparing a healthy breakfast for the morning and getting your clothes ready.

o   Enjoy a warm bath before bed especially if you add a couple of drops of lavender essential oil and/or some Epsom salts to aid muscle relaxation.

o   Get to bed by 10pm, and certainly before 11pm. Have a set time for bed and get up at the same time as this sleep routine helps the body have a stable circadian rhythm, which in turn means better quality and quantity of our sleep.

> If you are a shift worker, then please do visit a naturopath and/or acupuncturist to discuss ways to offset the sleep disruption you are experiencing.

## Foods for sleep

o   Eating late can affect the restorative action of sleep, leaving the digestion much to do instead of resting while we are sleeping. So eat dinner before 7pm if possible (at least two to three hours before bed).

o   Avoid a heavy evening meal. Try eating a big breakfast, a good lunch and a light, early dinner for ultimate digestive peace while you sleep.

o   Eat foods rich in magnesium to help relax your muscles - nuts and seeds, especially almonds and pumpkins seeds, dark green leafy vegetables, beans and pulses, yoghurt, avocado and banana.

o   Tryptophan-rich foods work in conjunction with melatonin to regulate and enhance sleep. This is why a warm glass of milk before bed can help some. Beef, turkey, eggs, legumes such as lentils, cottage cheese, dates, oats and bananas are other options. Nuts and seeds have tryptophan with the added value of magnesium and calcium to settle a frazzled nervous system and relax your muscles.

## Sleep promoters

o   Connection with your partner can be deeply relaxing for your body. Make time for each other in the evening for cuddles and intimacy, quiet heart to heart talking, expressing gratitude for each other, reciprocal massaging and touch, sharing a warm bath or slow walking outside together on a warmer night. If you're in the mood, sex can really help too.

o   Regular exercise (although avoided late at night i.e. not in the two hours before bed unless it's a gentle stretch or walk) will assist good, healthy sleep patterns.

o   Daily sunshine helps to regulate our body clock. A daily walk will work wonders, as will getting out in the sun as much as possible during the day (with sun safety in mind of course).

o   If you can't sleep, then try using progressive muscle relaxation by first tensing and then relaxing each area of the body. Breath in deeply, hold the contraction for three to five seconds then relax the muscles as you breathe out. Begin by contracting the muscles in the feet and work your way slowly up through your calves, thighs, buttocks, abdomen, chest, arms, shoulders, jaw, eyes, forehead and face. Feel the difference between the tense and relaxed muscles and you will find yourself letting go more and more. If your mind wanders, just gently bring your attention back to the next body part you were up to. If you get to your head and you are still awake, keep going, working your way from your head down to your feet.

o   If your mind is racing with thoughts about things you need to do tomorrow, it can really help to write them down. Sometimes the mind can obsess for fear of not remembering in the morning. Writing a list can help you to let it go until you can actually work on it in the morning.

o   If you are troubled or anxious then you may need to look at stress management tools (see more on this in Chapter 5) and taking up yoga, meditation or tai chi may be helpful.

o   Drinking good quality chamomile tea can improve sleep. Without being a sedative, its deeply relaxing qualities mean you get into deeply restful REM sleep quicker and stay in it for longer. It really takes the edge of anxiety too when consumed in good doses regularly. Use organic, loose leaf tea, make a big pot and drink 4-5 cups of hot or cold tea throughout the day for best effects. Try to avoid drinking before bed.

o   A five-minute routine of pre-bed stretching with slow, deep breathing can reduce cramping, restlessness and discomfort.

If you experience restless legs or regular calf or foot cramps in bed then it's time to consult a naturopath or nutritionist for advice as you may be low in magnesium, calcium or another nutrient.

o Cognitive behavioural therapy (CBT) is a psychotherapeutic approach, and research has indicated that it can be more effective than sleeping medication to treat chronic insomnia.[135] Contact your GP for a referral to a psychologist if you would like to try this approach.

o Download the Be Fertile CD – Guided Relaxations for your Sleep and listen nightly before sleep or if you wake in the night and can't easily return to sleep. There is a track on this album for general relaxation too. *www.befertile.com.au*

## Sleep disrupters

o Emails or social media browsing/posting in the hour before bed is too stimulating for getting to sleep easily. As well as being stimulating, screens are bright like sunlight and trick our body's rhythms to think we should be awake. Install a software program like *justgetflux.com* or *f.lux.com* which alter your computer screen as the evening progresses down to a soft warm glow, designed to help improve sleep. Even better, set your intentions to switch it all off at least one hour before your bed time and relax, read a print book instead or turn on some quiet music, chat, or enjoy cuddles and intimacy to wind down for sleep.

o Alcohol can also interrupt sleep and give the digestion and liver extra work that can hinder the repair that goes on when we sleep. While having a few drinks may help you to initially fall asleep, it hinders the body's ability to achieve deep, quality sleep. You are ideally avoiding it for best fertility outcomes, but if you do have a drink, notice how it affects you in all the ways you can't tell when you drink regularly. It will help your resolve to stay off it.

o   Sleeping pills may provide quick relief however, are not the best solution long-term as they become less effective and more addictive after only a few nights. They may also not be safe for your baby if you are trying to conceive. There are many herbal and nutritional options if extra help is needed to sort out your body clock but make sure you are getting the right dose with advice from a naturopath, herbalist or nutritionist.

> Other factors that adversely impact your sleep include pain, depression, anxiety, snoring and sleep apnoea. As these conditions may reduce the quality and quantity of your sleep, they are best addressed by seeking help from a health professional.

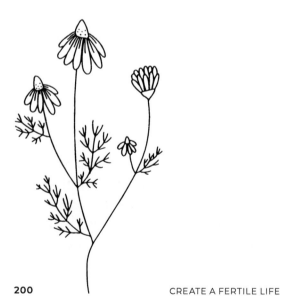

# TOP TIPS FOR HIM AND HER

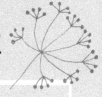

Aim for seven to nine hours' sleep daily.

Exercise, sunshine, meditation, journaling and talking
through problems can all help promote sleep quality.

Establish a peaceful bed time ritual and give attention
to creating a safe and lovely bedroom sanctuary
with a comfortable bed you can enjoy.

Saying no to caffeine drinks or foods will help enormously
to re-establish a good sleep pattern and reduce stress and
anxiety in your body too. If you do have it, try to keep it
before midday to minimise the effects on sleep..

Avoid eating after 7pm and aim to give alcohol a miss.

While sleep apnoea can affect women, it is more common
in men. If you are a profound snorer or fidgety sleeper,
a sleep check with your GP is a great idea.

No electronic devices in the bedroom including
TV's, laptops, tablets and mobile phones.

For chronic insomniacs you may need to go to your
doctor and request a referral to a psychologist
who specialises in CBT therapy.

# 7

# Building a safe environment for your fertility

In this chapter we are going to give you the basics around chemicals and radiation, but if you are interested in learning more about this (and really, everyone needs to) we recommend you read the report we talk about below (available free online) or read *Healthy Home, Healthy Family* by Melbourne-based building biologist, Nicole Bijlsma.[136]

---

## Nicole Bijlsma's Story

*After seven years of trying to conceive, Nicole's own challenging fertility issues drove her to become an expert in building biology, primarily to understand if and how her home might be negatively impacting on her chance of conceiving and carrying a healthy baby to full term. She was frustrated in their inability to start a family and she began to see how her health had declined after they moved into their home. Nicole suffered from poor sleep and fatigue initially, followed by a series of unexplained miscarriages.*

*After investigation, Nicole discovered that the previous couple living in their home had also had fertility problems. She found out their home was in a high-level magnetic field caused by the meter panel on the outside wall of their bed-head. Nicole diagnosed this consistent night time radiation exposure as the cause of her fatigue and insomnia since moving into their house, and a likely contributor to their fertility issues too.*

*During this time of learning about electromagnetic fields, chemicals in household products, and how to create a healthier home, they had sought help from a fertility specialist and underwent immune therapy. This resulted in pregnancy and their twins were born. When the twins were six months old the family moved to a new house. Before choosing their new rental home Nicole (by now an expert in the field of Building Biology) carefully assessed for electromagnetic fields, mould and geopathic stress.*

*Within two years of living in their new home, Nicole fell pregnant and this time needed no intervention to sustain a healthy pregnancy. She gave birth to their beautiful daughter Charlotte 9 months later.*

---

It may sound like an extreme comment, but it is true to say that every day we come into contact with a multitude of chemicals that are known – or at least heavily suspected – to cause cancer, infertility and birth defects. Every 60 seconds another twenty chemicals are registered for use on the world's largest database: The Chemical Abstract Service. Just to put that into context, that's 200,000 new chemicals every week, and over 143 million are currently registered for use as of July 2018.[137] Large population biomonitoring studies from across the globe have identified chemicals in humans from the womb to the tomb at levels known to cause adverse health effects. Of the man-made chemicals, over 80% of them have never been tested for their impact on human health as the burden of proof is not on industry to prove safety. Consequently, it takes years, decades, and even generations for researchers and governments to determine if a chemical is safe or hazardous. In 2006, the World Health Organisation's report on *State of the Science of Endocrine Disrupting Chemicals* 2012, highlighted the numerous chemicals in everyday products that impact on fertility, reproductive disorders, and are most significant for pregnant women and their unborn children.[138] It's a depressing read, and even more depressing is the general lack of response from both the media and governments to this warning.

It's not so extreme a view when you consider that the Danish government has launched several consumer campaigns on the negative impact of endocrine disrupting chemicals (EDCs) and have campaigned to warn pregnant women about the health impact on their unborn child - warning not to wear perfume, makeup, or use paints and pesticides. Denmark has also banned a number of chemicals used in food packaging.[139]

But, there is some good news. As individuals, we can educate ourselves around these exposure risks, and we have the power to decide — at least to a significant degree — the extent of our exposure. Until we do, most of us unknowingly bring these chemicals into our homes, put them on our skin, consume them in our food, and inhale them from solvents, plastics, pollution and cigarette smoke. There are alternatives — many in fact!

Although we are surrounded by these environmental hazards we can limit our exposure to them and we can also support our detoxification pathways to tirelessly eliminate this unwanted environmental load.

# WHAT IS SAFE?

It may surprise you to learn that less than 20% of the chemicals in consumer products have ever actually been tested for health effects according to the US Environmental Protection Agency. And when these toxicology studies do take place, exposure to only one chemical at a time is tested. But of course, we are exposed to dozens, even hundreds, of chemicals every day. Every chemical has the potential to interact and create different, even unexpected effects when combined with other chemicals. There is no research available to help us understand the effects of combined chemical exposure over time.

It is a common belief that everything stocked on the shelves in our supermarkets must be proven to be safe, and must have been tested. This is simply not true. These industries are self-regulated, and the research isn't there to show either short or long-term safety, especially when we're talking about fertility and pregnancy.

# HOW DOES THIS IMPACT MY FERTILITY?

The main concern with regard to fertility and the health of unborn children is the impact these chemicals have on our hormones. Many substances act as endocrine disruptors, meaning they disrupt the way your hormones work in your body. This is known to affect fertility in adults (sperm counts in men, oestrogen-dominant hormone conditions in women such as endometriosis, fibroids etc), reproductive development in unborn children (increasing the risks of malformed testes in male babies and future infertility in female babies), neuro-developmental disorders in unborn children, poorer egg numbers and fertilisation rates in women undergoing IVF and increased risks of pre-term birth for pregnant women.[139,140] Less significant but still concerning impacts include allergies and skin and lung irritation, especially for young children.

# 10-step guide to a more
# fertility friendly environment

These chemicals make their way into our homes and lives in varied ways when we don't know about or consider the impacts they may have. However if you follow our 10-step guide and make conscious choices to do things differently, you will significantly minimise your exposure, improving your health and fertility outcomes too. As an added bonus, you will be minimising many health risks into the future and improving the overall state of your family's health too.

## 1. AVOID THE USE OF PLASTICS WHEN STORING, PACKAGING, COOKING OR FREEZING FOOD AND AVOID CANNED FOODS.

Plastics used to package and store food as well as canned food (due to the plastic lining of the can) leach chemical compounds, many of which act as endocrine disruptors.

The most well recognised of these is bisphenol A (BPA), which researchers have confirmed works as an oestrogen disruptor, and can negatively affect both female and male fertility, as well as foetal development. Research has also shown that women with higher concentrations of BPA's in their bloodstream collected up to 24% fewer eggs on egg retrieval with IVF.[141] It is also alarming to note that BPA in the blood stream when pregnant with a boy will negatively impact his fertility later in life, with sperm concentration and motility significantly affected.[142]

While debate continues around whether or not BPA's should be banned from production, it remains one of the most ubiquitous chemicals in our homes and environment, and many of us would test positive if we were to check our blood concentrations at any time. Luckily, BPA's have a half-life of under 24 hours, and if we are conscious about our exposure, we can quickly limit their impact.

Whilst there are plenty of BPA free products on the market, these are not necessarily safe. Other plastics are also of concern, and the safest option is to limit exposure as much as possible.

## Food packaging and cooking utensils:

| ✗ WHAT TO AVOID | ✓ ALTERNATIVES |
|---|---|
| **Plastics** used to package and store food and drinks. | Purchase your food fresh, free of packaging, and store it only in paper, stainless steel or glass. This includes your water bottle, which should be glass or stainless steel. |
| **Tinned or canned foods** | If you can't cook/make your own, look for alternatives packaged in glass, or at a minimum, look for BPA free cans. |
| **Plastic cooking utensils** | When cooking, use only stainless steel, glass, and non-treated wooden utensils and appliances. |
| **Cling wrap** directly touching the food is especially problematic with high-fat content foods like cheese, meat, coconut cream, ice cream etc. | Store in paper, bees wax food wraps, jars, stainless steel or glass containers. Often glass containers have plastic lids. Wait until the food is cold before securing the lid and ensure the food is not touching the plastic. |

| ✗ WHAT TO AVOID | ✓ ALTERNATIVES |
|---|---|
| **Heating or freezing food in plastics**<br><br>Surprisingly, freezing food in plastics also encourages leaching of chemicals, and should be avoided.<br><br>Avoid microwaving (mostly due to potential radiation exposure) but if you do use it, never heat your food in plastic containers or with plastic wrap. | When heating, preferably use your stainless steel pots and heat over the stove; or use oven proof glass or suitable tray to heat in the oven. When freezing use glass containers. |

# 2. AVOID COMMERCIAL CLEANING PRODUCTS AND HOUSEHOLD 'HYGIENE' PRODUCTS

About 80% of ingredients in cleaning products have never been assessed for their impact on human health.

Manufacturers of cleaning products are not required by law to list their ingredients on the label, so it's often impossible to know what they contain. However, many fragrances and preservatives are known endocrine disruptors, which can impact your hormonal balance and thus affect your fertility. Instead, switch over to safer products and even better, make your own!

## Tips for cleaning with allergies and sensitivities:

The most effective way to reduce the allergen load in the home is with a damp microfibre cloth to dust the home and a suitable vacuum cleaner that is fitted with a HEPA (high efficiency particulate air) filter and motorised head. This will significantly reduce allergens like dust mites, pollens and pet dander. In addition, you should regularly open windows to promote fresh air, remove your shoes before you enter the home, and frequently air bedding and furnishings in the sun.

With regard to dealing with mould, tackling moisture is the key, so wipe showers with microfibre cloths immediately after bathing, install exhaust fans that vent the steam to the outside (not roof space), and dry any accidental water flows or plumbing leaks as soon as you become aware of them. To remove visible mould from grout, dip an old toothbrush into a mixture of bicarb soda and dish-liquid and scrub; if, however, the visible mould is in the silicone, you will need to replace it. If the visible mould exceeds the size of a piece of paper, or there's a damp, musty odour or history of water damage, contact a building biologist to assess the extent of the problem. This is especially important if any of the occupants suffer from asthma, allergies or chronic fatigue illnesses for which there is no obvious known cause.

| ✗ WHAT TO AVOID | ✓ ALTERNATIVES |
| --- | --- |
| **Cleaning products**<br><br>Bleach (commonly found in bathroom and floor cleaners).<br><br>Ammonia (oven and floor cleaners).<br><br>d-Limonene (orange-scented cleaning products).<br><br>'Fragrances' (often include known endocrine disruptors and petrochemicals) | A slightly damp micro-fibre cloth is effective at cleaning most surfaces. Dusting, windows, bench tops, tiles and walls can all effectively be cleaned by simply using these specialised cloths – no sprays, creams or chemicals needed!<br><br>**To reduce pathogenic bacteria:** Eucalyptus and tea tree oils are effective at killing over 99% of bacteria. Simply dilute 20 drops in a bucket of warm water, and use to mop your floors. Also great for cleaning and disinfecting toilets.<br><br>**For most kitchen and bathroom surfaces:** make a paste made of two parts bicarb soda to one part liquid detergent. This is also useful for cleaning your oven and stove top. Or for the kitchen sink sprinkle bicarb soda and drop some white vinegar over the top and scrub.<br><br>As far as we are aware the Abode cleaning products are the safest and cleanest available in Australia. |

| X WHAT TO AVOID | ✓ ALTERNATIVES |
|---|---|
| Household 'hygiene' products, such as anti-bacterials, air fresheners, scented rubbish bin bags, deodorisers and disinfectants. | Use essential oils to freshen the air e.g. orange oil, eucalyptus, tea tree etc. You can burn them or dilute a few drops in water and spray them around the room. Open the windows regularly for fresh air and try some leafy indoor plants to improve air quality. |

# 3. AVOID DRY CLEANING

The solvents used in dry cleaning are absorbed through the skin, and have been shown to negatively affect fertility.[143] They can be detected on the breath for up to 48 hours after you have worn the clothing.[144] If it is unavoidable to use a dry cleaner, then choose chemical-free dry cleaners, which are thankfully becoming more popular.

# 4. CHOOSE SAFER PERSONAL CARE PRODUCTS AND COSMETICS

Including shampoo and conditioner, hair care, skin care, sunscreens, make-up, perfumes and deodorants.

> It is estimated that the average woman has applied 126 different chemicals in 12 different products to her face, body and hair before she even leaves the house for the day.

Australian women are exposed to an average of 160 chemicals per day from their personal care products, and for men it's around half of that. When you learn that less than half of these products have been tested for safety, and never been tested for their combined impact, that is a worrying statistic.

## The effects of personal care products on pregnancy

Recent research shows that women exposed to higher levels of the chemical compound, called phthalates, through normal everyday exposure (found in shampoos, detergents, cosmetics and soft plastics) were up to five times more likely to experience premature delivery, which the researchers noted had increased in incidence in developed countries in the past two decades.[145] In the past few years, phthalates have also been linked to asthma, ADHD, breast cancer, obesity, Type 2 diabetes, low IQ, neurodevelopmental and behavioural issues, autism spectrum disorders, altered reproductive development and male fertility issues.

| ✕ WHAT TO AVOID | ✓ ALTERNATIVES |
| --- | --- |
| Commercial shampoo, conditioner, body wash, hair gel, hair spray, skin care, sunscreens, makeup (especially tinted lipstick), nail polish, perfumes, fragrances and deodorants. | Consult the website set up by the American Environmental Working Group on this subject: *www.ewg.org/skindeep*. <br><br> Also a book and app called *The Chemical Maze www.chemicalmaze.com*. <br><br> You can look up the products you're using (most Australian products are listed too) and easily see their rating of the potential toxic risk of that product. Look for "phthalate-free" on the label. |
| Hair dye. | Use natural dyes, henna or consider highlighting your hair instead so that your scalp is not exposed to the chemicals. |

| ✗ WHAT TO AVOID | ✓ ALTERNATIVES |
|---|---|
| Regular sunscreen. | Choose a natural sunscreen or a fertility-friendly sunscreen that may use zinc oxide, which sits on top of the skin. |
| | Cover up with long sleeves and hats and sit in the shade to avoid over use of sunscreens. |
| | Consult the Environmental working group guide to sunscreens at *www.ewg.org/2015sunscreen* |

Of course, we're not recommending you start walking around looking and smelling as if you just climbed out of a cave, but we do recommend you choose these products carefully, as some are better than others. If you've got eight minutes and want to learn more about this, you can view The Story of Cosmetics (2010) on YouTube.[146]

# 5. WHEN POSSIBLE, AVOID RENOVATIONS AND IF PURCHASING NEW FURNITURE, CHECK FOR NON-TOXIC MATERIALS

That new car/renovation smell is actually the release of hormone-disrupting chemicals. If you are planning on building, renovating or buying a new car, home or furniture, please check *Healthy Home, Healthy Family* as a guide or the web site *www.buildingbiology.com. au* before you do so. It's natural to want to renovate in preparation for a new family and we often find couples mid-renovation when they see us. We recommend either delay the renovation, or if you do renovate please look for non-toxic materials and move out while the work is being undertaken. Wear protective clothing and gear (ie quality masks, gloves etc) if you are doing any handy work your self.

# 6. AVOID SOURCES OF MERCURY INCLUDING MERCURY DENTAL FILLINGS (AMALGAMS) AND EATING LARGE FISH

Dental amalgams are a common source of mercury exposure and the older the filling, the more likely it is to be releasing mercury fumes. Mercury is a hazardous metal known to irreversibly damage neurodevelopment in unborn babies. During a pre-conception time or when you are trying to conceive is not the ideal time to replace any mercury amalgams as that might expose you to a higher load. Eat a diet high in antioxidant fruits and vegetables to help protect cells against any heavy metals including mercury.

However, our major source of exposure to mercury is though our food chains. Sadly, we have polluted our oceans with the toxic waste products of industry, and hence we have poisoned our fish and our food. Mercury concentrations are higher in large fish that eat other smaller fish, as accumulation occurs up the food chain. Notably, this includes tuna, shark (flake) and swordfish. For a full list of fish to avoid, check out details in Chapter 9, Step 5.

# 7. AVOID EXPOSURE TO HEAVY METALS WHERE POSSIBLE

Lead is another hazardous metal known to irreversibly damage neurodevelopment in unborn babies. Lead was removed from our petrol late last century, and as a result exposure levels have luckily plummeted. But it is still worth noting a number of concerning areas in which exposure may occur.

All surfaces painted prior to the 1980s will contain up to 90% lead-based paints. When undisturbed, this causes no problems. But when the paint flakes or is removed and turned to dust, problems arise.

When renovating or re-painting, it is very important to ensure you are not exposing yourself to these particles, which can easily be breathed in. We recommend either leaving the paint on the wall and painting over it, or employing professionals, such as The Lead Group (*www.lead.org.au*) or the Australian Dust Removalists Association (*www.adra.com.au*), who will ensure that all traces of lead dust are safely removed from your home.

**Did you know that your lipstick may contain lead?**

Sadly, up to 80% of tinted lipsticks contain lead. This is not some great conspiracy by the cosmetic industry to poison women with a well-known neurotoxic heavy metal, but simply a result of the use of pigments mined from the earth, which naturally contain lead. Unless each and every batch is tested, lead concentrations cannot be confirmed, and therefore the best advice is to avoid or minimise the use of coloured lipsticks, at least when trying to conceive and when pregnant.

**Avoid anti-perspirants, antacids, aluminium tin cans and other sources of aluminium**

Aluminium is another toxic metal that we often come into contact with that may have an effect on fertility and the unborn child. It is thought to have a detrimental effect on our brain function and it may compromise our nutritional status.

Aluminium is found in anti-perspirants, so choose a natural deodorant instead. Most antacids contain significant amounts of this substance so if reflux is a problem discuss this with your naturopath or TCM practitioner for natural support with herbs and dietary suggestions. Beer and soft drink cans are made from aluminium and some of the metal will be leeched into these drinks. Both beer and soft drinks are on our list of drinks to avoid for optimal fertility, so this is another reason to take that message on board.

If you are concerned about your potential heavy-metal exposure in the past, consult your naturopath regarding a hair-mineral analysis to identify any issues.

**Sources of aluminium to avoid:**

o   Anti-perspirants.

o   Antacids.

o   Beer and soft drink cans.

o   Aluminium foil.

o   Old aluminium cookware.

o   Baking powders.

o   Common table salt.

# 8. FILTER YOUR DRINKING WATER AND AVOID BOTTLED WATER

Water is a controversial topic. It is commonly said that in Australia we 'have some of the cleanest drinking water in the world', but that really depends on how you define the term 'clean'. If you are referring to bacteria, yes absolutely, most of our drinking water is clean. But if you are referring to contamination by heavy metals and pesticides, or the addition of chemicals highly suspect in contributing to various types of cancer, then sadly no, our water is not ideal.

Heavy metals leach into our water supply from the pipes it travels through to reach our houses, and most significantly, from the pipes between the water mains and our taps, especially if your plumbing is old. Aluminium, lead and copper are commonly found in household tap water. Aluminium and lead are known to be neurotoxic, and unborn babies and infants are most at risk. Copper toxicity significantly compromises your zinc levels, and this copper-to-zinc ratio is essential for effective hormone production and supporting a healthy pregnancy.

Pesticides are not regularly tested in our water supply, and the concentration will depend heavily on the environment of our water sources. Simple tests can be purchased to determine if your water contains pesticides and heavy metals. Type 'watersafe test kits' into your search engine if you are concerned.

Chlorine, added to our water supply to kill bacteria is suspected of increasing the risk of bladder and kidney disease, and also for being responsible for damaging the healthy bacteria in our gut.[136] It's also a strong skin, lung and eye irritant, and is responsible for the exacerbation of symptoms many eczema sufferers experience after a shower. Some chlorine will evaporate when water is boiled or left in an open container for 24 hours.

Fluoride competes with iodine for uptake by the thyroid gland, and may exacerbate thyroid disorders in susceptible individuals. It is worth noting that fluoride is known to assist in preventing tooth decay when it comes into contact with teeth but has absolutely no benefit when ingested. We recommend at the very least you avoid fluoride in your drinking water if you have been diagnosed with or have a family history of thyroid problems.

Filtering your tap water is important if you are concerned about any of the above issues. This is also a complex debate, as different filters remove different substances. All will remove bacteria (unless the filters themselves have not been cleaned), and most will remove heavy metals and chlorine. Fluoride requires specific forms of filtration, such as reverse osmosis. With water filters, as with most things in life, you get what you pay for.

## Tips on choosing a water filter

Simply put, reverse osmosis is best when it comes to filtering our water as it removes fluoride and other chemicals and bacteria, but practically this can be difficult as it's expensive and it strips the water of the good minerals too. Next best thing is much more affordable carbon-block filters, which are readily available. We recommend the dual under sink filters.

Bottled water may also be of concern. To start with, all water bottled in plastic should be avoided, and be aware there are few regulations regarding the quality of bottled water in Australia and that there is nothing stopping companies from using filtered and even unfiltered tap water (which simply means you are paying about 2000 times more for the same quality of water). It is also legal for companies to add fluoride to bottled water. If you are going to buy water, please choose water in glass bottles or non-plastic casks. Check the label to ensure it is natural spring water and no fluoride has been added.

See the following website for more details on choosing the right water filter for your needs *(www.buildingbiology.com.au).*[147]

# 9. DON'T FORGET THAT YOUR FOOD HAS PESTICIDES TOO!

Unless we are always eating organic food, every time we have a meal we are ingesting pesticides or insecticides. Our fruit and vegetables and other crops can be sprayed many times before reaching our plate and these sprays are designed to damage or at least impair the reproduction of organisms. This is how they work to kill bugs and bacteria, but our bodies are made of billions of individual cells and organisms, that are individually susceptible to this damage. When it comes to fertility we're often talking about the health of individual cells, so minimising exposure can be particularly relevant if you're having trouble conceiving. That's why we suggest you choose organic foods as much as possible.

# 10. REDUCE YOUR EXPOSURE TO RADIATION

Our bodies are exposed to natural sources of radiation every day through sunshine and from the earth. The problem develops from our chronic exposure to man-made radiation from modern technologies such as mobile phones, laptops, Wi-Fi and microwave ovens. Radiation exposure is difficult to assess, as you can't see it, feel it, smell it or hear it. But we know it's there, and these days – more often than not – we're exposed to some form of radiation for most of the day and night, at unprecedented levels that are ever-increasing with the exponential growth in wireless technologies.

To understand why radiation is a problem, it's important to know exactly what the adverse effects of exposure can be. Ionising radiation damages the DNA bonds in cells, leading to chromosomal abnormalities or cell death. Non-ionising radiation can cause thermal heating (and potentially burning) via induced currents and electron excitation. When we are talking about fertility, nothing is as important as cellular health and DNA structure. As discussed in the Introduction to this book, successful conception depends on the delivery of 23 perfect chromosomes from each the sperm and the egg, to create the potential for an entire healthy human to be made. Sperm, in particular, are very small, delicate and susceptible cells, and they are especially vulnerable to the effects of radiation, thermal and non-thermal effects and direct heat from the same sources. It is entirely possible that radiation exposure is responsible for many incidences of male infertility and unexplained infertility.

While there is considerable debate on this, the scientific community agrees that more research is needed to further our understanding. In 2011, the International Agency for Research on Cancer (IARC) from the World Health Organization (WHO) released a statement adding radiofrequency electromagnetic fields (including microwave and millimeter waves) to their list of factors which are possibly carcinogenic to humans.

The good news is that most of the time, a matter of metres will change your exposure from extreme to negligible, so be aware that simply creating space between you and your radiation source of approximately two metres will reduce the impact.

**What type of radiation is the most problematic?**

| MOST DAMAGING | MODERATELY DAMAGING |
|---|---|
| Ionising radiation | Non-ionising radiation |
| o X-rays<br>o Gamma rays<br>o 'Cosmic radiation' found in the Earth's atmosphere and the radiation we are exposed to when flying. | o Microwaves and millimeter waves such as mobile phones, laptops, tablets, computers, Wi-Fi, microwave ovens, radio and satellite communications, radars, airport scanners, 4G and 5G networks, smart meters and other wireless or bluetooth devices etc.<br>o Radio waves such as broadcasting, radio communication, radar and other navigation systems, computer networks etc.<br>o Infrared, visible and UV light.<br>o Electricity sources such as power lines and cables, appliances such as electric blankets, hair driers, television, clock radios (even in standby mode). |

All of these are less damaging than ionizing radiation, but far more prevalent in our day to day lives.

Probably the most consistent concerns as far as day-to-day exposure goes are mobile phones and laptop computers or tablets. It is also important to consider your proximity to mobile phone towers, smart meters, Wi-Fi devices, routers, modems, Bluetooth devices such as printers, headsets, wireless keyboards, mouses, photocopiers, cordless phones, remote controls, microwave ovens and more.

As well as keeping your devices out of your pocket/bra/lap and away from your body at more than arm's length where possible, think about switching off wherever you can too. It may seem extreme, but it is the best way to reduce your exposure. Think about when you put your phone on silent, you're driving, socializing, watching a movie or other times when you won't be answering/responding anyway - why not just turn it to flight mode? What about when you are at your computer but not accessing the Internet? Or not at your computer at all? Might as well turn off your Wi-Fi connection and even your modem. If you are watching a movie, download it and turn off the Wi-Fi. Or when your battery is full, unplug it from the power. We can't control much of what is around us from mobile phone towers, modems and even our friends or colleagues' devices, but if we can switch our own devices off, we will reduce some exposure.

## Are your sperm being fried?

Fellas, there is now some evidence that carrying your mobile phone in your pocket damages sperm health.[148] Research presented at the American Society for Reproductive Medicine meeting in 2007 found that men who use cell phones for 4 hours a day had a 25% lower sperm count than those who don't use cell phones. Of the sperm they did have, 80% were not properly formed, and motility (a measure of swimming ability and a crucial factor in conception) was down by a third.

Similarly, research has shown that sperm exposed to a laptop computer connected to Wi-Fi is compromised within hours.[149] While researchers don't yet know why, the best advice is simply to not carry your phone in your pocket, and if you have to, turn it onto flight mode. Whenever you are sitting, make sure your phone is at least an arms-length reach away from you or further. When using a laptop, don't sit it on your lap. Distance is the key and remember to get in the habit of switching off your devices from Wi-Fi whenever possible.

Of course, the other regular exposure we often see is from air travel. If you are having trouble conceiving or have experienced miscarriage, your best bet is to minimise your time in the air, or to avoid it all together for three months prior to conception and for at least the first twelve weeks of pregnancy. Also consult with your naturopath regarding suitable antioxidants and supplements to support your body to cope with the effects of flying.

## How to reduce your radiation exposure when flying

Here are a few steps you can take if you have an unavoidable flight:

- Choose an aisle or middle seat (away from the window) as this may help reduce your radiation exposure.

- Don't drink alcohol – your liver needs all the help it can get to process the increase in radiation exposure.

- Keep you water intake up to support effective detoxification pathways. Take your own teabag and ask the flight attendant for a cup of (usually free!) hot water. Try antioxidant rich green tea or rooibos or to support detoxification pathways try dandelion root or chai.

- Pack antioxidant rich foods with colourful or dark green vegetable and fruits rather than relying on in-flight meals. For snacks, try some dark chocolate, berries, purple grapes, goji berries, pecans or Brazil nuts.

- Take a few sachets of spirulina or chlorella to drink every four to six hours on the flight. It is nutrient and antioxidant rich and a great detox superfood.

- Investigate anti-radiation blankets, belly bands, boxer shorts or protective clothing. They are soft cotton embedded with silver fiber to reflect radiation and minimise exposure to the body.

- It has been said that soaking in a bath with two cups of Epsom salts will assist your body to detox any radiation. While there isn't any research to support this, a long soak in a bath after a long-haul flight never hurt anyone! This would be best enjoyed before bedtime in your new time zone to help you have a more restful sleep and minimise jet lag. If you are pregnant, avoid a hot bath and and ensure the bath is only warm.

## How to reduce your exposure to radiation in your bedroom

The impact of radiation exposure is cumulative, so it's worth putting in some effort to achieve a radiation 'detox' every day. The easiest time for this tends to be at night when we are sleeping and will give us 7-9 hours of radiation-free time every day. This is conveniently also the most important time to be free of radiation, as your immune system and liver are busy repairing and detoxing your body during this window.

- Check your bedroom for electrical appliances and ensure anything within two metres of your bed is either moved away or turned off at the wall when sleeping (including lamps, clock radios, electric blankets, televisions, computers, mobile phones etc).

o   Check your smart meter/fuse box: if it's within three metres of where you sleep, move the bed! This may sound extreme, but the effects of the exposure to this cyclic radiation are potentially very significant, and we regularly see dramatic improvements in sleep quality when this issue is identified and rectified.

o   Check any other appliances that may be on the other side of your bedroom wall, whether it be your own home, or a wall shared with neighbours.

o   Make your home a jungle! Many plants have the ability to help detoxify air pollutants and radiation. Specific plants such as the Spider plant, Golden pothos, Peace lily, Chinese evergreen, Aloe vera, Gerbera daisy, Chrysanthemum, English ivy, Snake plant, Rhapis palm and Areca palm can act as air filtering plants.[150]

For extra motivation to follow our tips, hire a radiation detection device and try it around your home and workplace. You can see for yourself the difference it makes when you put your phone to flight mode, turn off your Wi-Fi or close your computer. You will also see which rooms of the house are relatively free from radiation emissions compared with others, so you can make choices about where you spend most of the time, and perhaps consider moving your bed, desk or couch.

# TOP TIPS FOR HIM AND HER

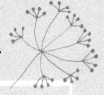

Minimise exposure to endocrine disrupting plastics
by removing them from everyday use in your
kitchen (including BPA lined canned foods).

Go to your cupboards right now and throw out all those toxic
cleaners! Look out for environmentally-friendly cleaning
products (www.cleanabode.com.au), or make your own!

Find your nearest chemical-free dry cleaner, and
consider making the shift. You'll notice as soon as
you enter the shop, they smell far less toxic compared
to your conventional cleaners.

Make the change to natural personal care products,
including deodorants, skin & hair care and cosmetics. There
are so many options out there, and natural products are
often far more beautiful to touch and beneficial for your skin.
Check out Skin Deep or Chemical Maze websites for more
info (*www.ewg.org/skindeep www.chemicalmaze.com*)

We understand that this one is huge for a lot of you, but
if your renovation or new furniture can wait, put it off,
especially while you could be pregnant. If not, consider
moving out while the work is being completed.

# TOP TIPS FOR HIM AND HER

Avoid mercury exposure by eliminating suspect seafood (for a full list of fish to avoid, check Chapter 9), and by ensuring your amalgam fillings are NOT removed during the preconception window or during pregnancy.

Be aware of other potential heavy metal sources (lead, aluminium) and avoid as much as possible. If you are concerned about your history of potential heavy metal exposures, speak to your naturopath about testing.

Get yourself a glass or stainless-steel water bottle, and drink 1.5-3 litres of clean filtered water from a recommended source each day.

Choose organic wherever possible for all of your food and personal care products.

Reduce radiation by simple things such as choosing to not carry your phone in your pocket and not resting your computer or tablet on your lap. Give yourself a two meter radiation exclusion zone while you sleep. Switch off your Wi-Fi, turn your phone to flight mode and remove all electronics from your bedroom. Fill your rooms with plants that can help detoxify radiation and filter the air in our home. What a beautiful way to benefit your health and even your fertility!

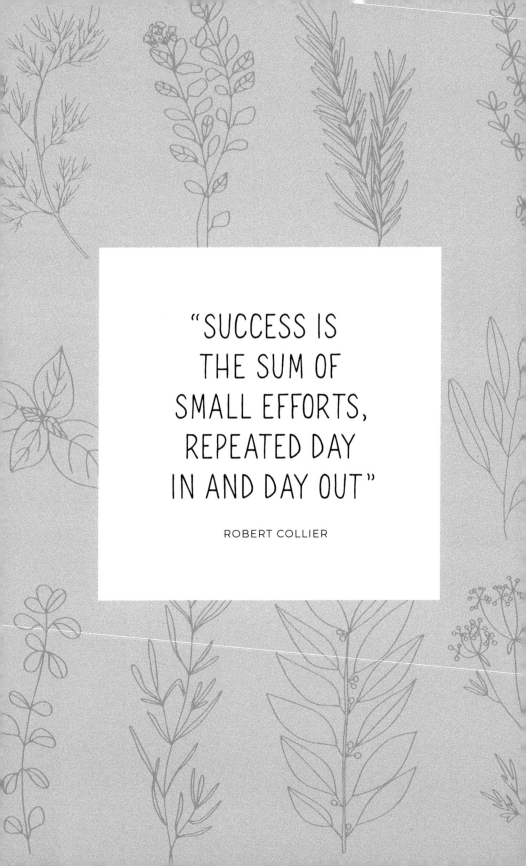

"SUCCESS IS
THE SUM OF
SMALL EFFORTS,
REPEATED DAY
IN AND DAY OUT"

ROBERT COLLIER

PART TWO

# **Feed**
## Your fertility diet

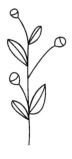

# IN THIS SECTION:

# 8

# Why change your eating habits to enhance your fertile potential?

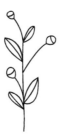

*M*y alarm goes off in the morning and I hit snooze and roll over. Ahhhh! Time to get up! If I hit the snooze button I will get an extra five minutes in bed... yes that's what I need... if I skip breakfast, then that means another 10 minutes lie in. I'll just have a hot drink and a muffin when I get to work instead.*

*Lunchtime rolls around and I haven't prepared anything (that was my sleep-in time). I pick up something at the cafe next to work. They don't have a great range but I grab a ciabatta with ham and cheese, which will keep me going.*

*Mid-afternoon, my energy levels are dropping — how will I will get through until knock-off time? I pop into the work kitchen and there is some left-over birthday cake from the boss's celebration yesterday... One piece will give me the boost I need to get through till 5pm.*

*Finally, the day is over and I grab my bags and run for the train.*
*Wouldn't you know it, my train has been cancelled. I am starving.*
*I grab a chocolate bar from the nearby machine to tide me over.*
*By the time I get home, I'm exhausted and so hungry I could eat*
*the entire contents of the pantry. What am I going to cook for dinner?*
*I need to eat now. Where's that phone number for Uber delivery?*

Life is busy and sometimes it is just really hard to balance everything and often our diet can 'go out the window'. It can be hard to eat well when we are tired or time-poor but there has never been a more important reason why you need to do as much as possible to get your diet on the straight and narrow; you are trying to make a baby!

## WHAT TO EAT AND WHY

Let's get into it! We will cover everything from our general day-to-day fertility diet, to superfoods, antioxidants, the specifics for egg and sperm health and much, much more! This will help you understand what to eat and, most importantly, why! We believe that if you understand why good food is so important, you are much more likely to feel inspired to eat it. Knowing that simple foods can make a big impact on your health and fertility is really inspiring. After all, what else do you do as frequently as eat? There aren't many things, which is why it is so important to get this right. There are plenty of researchers who have confirmed the importance of healthy eating to improve your chance of conceiving.[7,8,151–153] No one approach will fit everybody but after reading this section, you will be clear about what approach you need to improve your fertility through food.

## YOU ARE WHAT YOU EAT

What's your take on the saying 'you are what you eat'? How literal do you feel it is? We suspect that people shrug it off – after all, none of us are walking around actually looking like a piece of steak, or a chick pea or a banana! Yet, this saying is one of the wisest and best that we know. We are, quite literally, made from what we eat. Far from simply being fuel for our bodies like the petrol we put in our car, our bodies are made up only of the things we put into it (and a few things it can make up on its own based on what we put in). Our bodies are incredibly clever, because even if we don't put the perfect thing in, our super-smart engineering will try to make do with what it is given. This means we have a very high tolerance for the wrong kind of fuel, but eventually it will take a toll on our engines.

While food does provide us with energy — fuel for our body to function and be active — it provides so much more! When you put petrol in your car it is burned up in combustion, which propels pistons that makes things move, propels the car forward and does not contribute to the 'body' of the car at all. The human body is completely different. Food is broken down into highly-specialised components: stuff that is burned quickly for energy production, stuff that is stored to use as energy later on and a whole host of microscopic elements that are the very building blocks of our physical bodies — protein for our muscles, fats for our cells, nervous system, eyes and brain, iron for our blood, calcium and magnesium to make our bones and help our muscles and nervous system function and so much more. It is not enough simply to get calories (petrol) for our engine, we need a wide range of nutrients to perform very specific functions to maintain a vital body capable of health, healing, reproduction and longevity.

Without overwhelming you with science, let's just talk about one little element to demonstrate the 'you-are-what-you-eat' principle — the membranes of our cells. The inner and outer layers are made up essentially of fatty acids. The fatty membrane surrounding it provides the cell with shape and integrity, protecting it from infiltration from undesirables, facilitating the transport of nutrients into, and wastes out of the cell, and providing the main messenger system for our hormones to 'talk' to the cells. A lack of integrity in the fatty layer means the immunity of that cell is compromised as things may pass into the cell unchecked and unregulated and impact on the hormonal messages required to tell the cells how to act, putting the cell, and your health at risk.

Our bodies construct the fatty outer membranes of our cells from essential fatty acids found in foods we consume (in this case 'essential' means the body cannot make its own). Foods that contain these good fat sources include nuts and seeds, fish, avocado, coconut and more (see Chapter 9 for more about foods containing essential fatty acids.) Cell membranes can be damaged in many ways, but one of these is by not supplying adequate nutrition for the body to furnish cells with a healthy membrane, resulting in poor cell function, compromised immunity and even risk of cell death.

## OPTIMISING YOUR BABY'S HEALTH

So really think about this. Your baby will start out as two single cells, an egg and a sperm, coming together to form a fertilised egg – your embryo. It will then go through a rapid process of cell division which, if successful, over the next 40 weeks will develop into the very complex being that will be your baby. This incredibly rapid development and cell division is the fastest and most complex development we go through in our entire lives. We go from one cell of essential information (DNA), to becoming a complex human with a brain, eyes, hearing, skin, organs, a nervous system, blood, bone marrow, emotions and so much more. This is absolutely miraculous, beautiful, and mystifying!

But why does this matter? Firstly, the little fertilised egg needs all the help it can get if it is going to make it all the way through to the many trillions of cells it will eventually become. It needs to be strong, healthy, vital and protected. To function properly, it needs to be made up of enough essential fatty acids to form a strong lipid bilayer, which will form its protective outer layer. If the cell membrane is not well formed, its survival is at risk. And this is just one of the risks this little egg faces on the intense journey forward from here. This is your potential baby we are talking about.

Problems arise when we eat too much of the wrong kind of fats. In particular, trans-fats from processed, fried and convenience foods that have poor nutritional value. They do not function in the body in the ways healthy fats do; they create inflammation, cardiovascular disease and compromised reproductive health. Trans-fats do damage while healthy fats perform essential functions and maintain health. Recent research has even shown that people who eat fast food four or more times a week are less likely to conceive within one year and increases the chance of infertility from 8% to 16%.[154]

Healthy fats affect the proper functioning of not only your cells, but also your hormones, skin, eyes, nervous system, brain, blood, bowel function – it is almost endless. Additionally, we are only talking about one nutrient here! We could go on and on about the ways in which various nutrients act in our bodies but as a start, this illustrates the point neatly. Your body needs you to eat well in order to maintain health, vitality, function, survival and, of course, reproduction.

Nature does not want to reproduce shabby cells, so our bodies have ways of identifying and eliminating them. Eating well ensures this function works adequately to protect us from harm. It also means that when it comes to reproducing a new human, those early cells are up to mother nature's exacting standards and aren't discarded for not coming up to scratch.

Without a doubt, food provides the foundation for creating and sustaining life and health. Many patients talk about their desire to use food as medicine and it most certainly is the best approach. However, while this foundation is absolutely essential, in many cases it is often not enough. People who are depleted of essential nutrients may find it difficult to repair a deep deficiency through eating alone. For example, it can be difficult for a menstruating woman to repair a long-standing iron deficiency while she continues to lose blood every month. This is particularly true if there is any menstrual pathology causing heavy bleeding (think endometriosis or fibroids) or if she is a vegetarian, vegan or eating a predominantly plant based diet.

Some people need to supplement their diet. In our experience, the reality is that not many people are really eating enough of the vital foods to ensure adequate nutrition from food alone. If you eat cereal from a box, shop predominantly at the supermarket, eat processed, junk or takeaway foods regularly and consume alcohol, coffee or sugar regularly, then you probably can't claim to be using food as medicine.

## OPTIMISING YOUR FERTILITY – BUT THERE IS MORE!

In most cases it is not enough to have merely adequate nutrition. For optimal fertility in particular, replete nutrient levels are required – this means well established high levels of essential nutrients, particularly essential fatty acids, folate, vitamin D, iodine, B-vitamins, vitamins A and E, iron, selenium, zinc, coenzyme Q10, calcium, magnesium and more. Many of the essential vitamins, minerals, plant compounds and macronutrients, such as protein, fats and carbohydrates, are needed for multiple functions. Our bodies have an intelligent hierarchy, and essential organs such as the heart and brain will benefit from important nutrients first. This means that if we are not fully replete in vital nutrients, our reproduction will be one of the body systems to suffer, under-function and be a possible cause of sub-fertility.

If a pregnancy occurs, nutrient requirements increase immediately. In fact, pregnant and breastfeeding women have the highest nutritional requirements of anyone – the highest of their entire life.

That is a pretty amazing and telling fact. They are creating a body and that body is made up of vitamins, minerals, fats, protein and carbohydrates from the food a pregnant woman eats.

We have already discussed how much rapid development is happening in early pregnancy and we know that many women find eating difficult due to nausea in the first trimester. More than enough is the only way to ensure that enough is enough when it comes to preparing for pregnancy!

If your nutritional levels are borderline at the time of conception, they can quickly drop to inadequate levels in early pregnancy, putting a developing foetus at risk. If nutrition is inadequate, the cell may not have what it needs to go the distance. Coenzyme Q10 (CoQ10) is a great example of this, and one of those nutrients that declines in our bodies with age. Among the various functions of this nutrient is provision of fuel for cells. CoQ10 provides the basic fuel for the engine within the cell (the mitochondria) to produce energy (adenosine triphosphate or ATP). This is especially important if IVF is required. Once a cell is taken from the body, it only has its own resources to keep it going. Adequate levels of CoQ10 in the embryo help to ensure that tiny cell engine has enough fuel to keep going on its own until it is returned to the body as an embryo, where Mum's metabolism will take over again. Once again, isn't our body just miraculous? We truly marvel when we think about this divine cleverness!

**We are all different. Some of us are like weeds in the footpath that will survive and thrive no matter what life and the environment throw at us. Others are more like a rare orchid or prize rose bush requiring high maintenance: just the right amounts of sunlight, moisture and compost and even then will only bloom in the damp night air of the full moon in June. Being kind to ourselves, understanding our physical, mental and emotional needs, and ensuring they are fulfilled is the best basis for anyone to begin from.**

# TOP TIPS FOR HIM AND HER

Simple foods can make a big impact on your health
and fertility. There is plenty of research to show
the importance of healthy eating to improve your
chance of conceiving.

Eat healthy fats and avoid the wrong kind of
fats, in particular trans-fats from processed,
fried and convenience foods.

We are what we eat and eating well ensures our cells
reproduce in healthy ways and can reproduce a new human.

A healthy balanced diet is the foundation to create
a fertile life; however, be aware you may need more
if you have nutritional deficiencies.

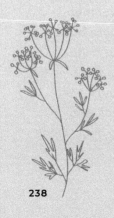

CREATE A FERTILE LIFE

# 9

# Eating for fertility

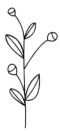

There is no one dietary approach that will suit everyone. However, there are some general principles that apply to all and then some specific tweaks for particular conditions, body-types, or special needs. We will cover all of that here. This is a big section so be sure to plough through it – you only need to get this information once to be able to thoroughly overhaul your approach to food, or at the very least, make the specific adjustments you need for your condition or stage.

Most importantly, everyone could do with getting out of their food box and stretching their imagination and scope for eating a truly broad and colourful diet rich with variety. Because we need to eat three times a day we can get lazy – skipping meals, especially the all-important breakfast, eating the same old thing day-in, day-out, picking up some take-away when we can't be bothered, eating on the run or while working, or just not making great choices – every meal counts! All impact on our health and, over time, can really leave us feeling pretty low on energy and vitality.

Start by working your way through the top eight recommendations towards a more fertile diet. As you incorporate each one, tick them off and move onto the next. For example, you may recognise that you don't eat the recommended intake of five serves (approximately three cups) of vegetables a day; so you may choose to start off by working on attending to this.

# **8 steps** to a more fertile diet

## 1. EAT AT LEAST THREE CUPS OF VEGETABLES EVERY DAY

All vegetables contain a great range of nutrients important for your health, however, from a fertility point of view we really want to see lots more of the green leafy family, including silverbeet, spinach, rocket, kale, lettuce, parsley, coriander, mint, etc. They are essential for women who are preparing for pregnancy or are pregnant as they contain folate in a highly absorbable form. These foods are a good source of fibre as well as being high in important vitamins B, C, and K as well as beta carotene, the pregnancy safe precursor to Vitamin A. Maximise your daily intake with a green smoothie, big green salad or steamed with dinner.

### Tips to get more vegetables:

o Add some to your breakfast! Throw in a mix of vegetables (e.g. mushrooms, baby spinach, rainbow chard or kale etc) into an omelette or stirfry and serve with poached/boiled eggs.

o Snack on veggies. Cut up some carrot, celery, cucumber, red capsicum and cherry tomatoes, and nibble on these mid-morning or afternoon. They are even better when dipped into some yummy hummus, tzatziki or avocado dip, or spread with some nut butter (almond nut butter on celery is a delicious combination).

- Add some veggies to your smoothie. A big handful of baby spinach, lettuce leaves, rocket, avocado or cucumber are easy to throw into a daily smoothie.

- Have stir fries for dinner: an easy dish to load with veggies.

- Grate up veggies and cook them into your sauces, e.g. load your bolognese with carrots, celery and zucchini. Serve your pasta sauce on steamed broccolini, string beans or asparagus, or use a zucchini spiroli instead of pasta.

- Get in the habit of making big green salads with lots of different herbs and lettuce types, Chinese broccoli, celery, spring onions or chives, raw broccolini etc. It is nice to chop everything down quite small, make a big blend, and coat in a simple lemon and extra virgin olive oil dressing.

- Blitz up some homemade dips e.g. blend some butter beans, fresh coriander, garlic, lemon juice, olive oil and a handful of baby spinach and herbs like dill or coriander to make a yummy dip that is great to have with your meals or as a snack.

- Blend a green sauce to have on everything! Load your blender with uncooked leafy herbs (try dill, coriander, parsley), garlic, olives, lemon juice or preserved lemons and a big glug of extra virgin olive oil. Have this on baked veggies, fish or red meat or on a rice or corn cake or toasted seed bread as a snack. Experiment with different combinations.

Once you are on top of this then take it one step further and eat a rainbow every day. Sounds good, huh? By this we mean, think about the food you are putting on your plate and aim to eat as many colours as you can each day. Colours in your foods come mainly from vegetables and fruits and of course these should make up the majority of your diet – vegetables in particular. That means thinking up creative ways of getting colour into breakfast, lunch and dinner, which actually isn't that hard: think blueberries and strawberries with breakfast, a salad of greens, beetroot, capsicum and squash with lunch and a stir fry of chick peas, cauliflower, broccoli, corn, carrots and fresh herbs for dinner.

## How does my fertility benefit if I eat the rainbow?

A colourful diet will ensure you get plenty of micronutrients (vitamins and minerals), phytochemicals (helpful plant food compounds), plus the all-important antioxidants needed in your body every day – all of which are essential for optimal fertility.

Antioxidants within our body and in our diet have the job of dealing with free radicals and reactive oxygen species (both are categories of common damaging substances), which can be implicated in cell damage including damage to our eggs and sperm. In fact, low levels of antioxidants have also been linked to recurrent miscarriage. The free radical load is increased by many things in our environment and in our food, including:

- o Pesticides (exposure through foods and environment).
- o Smoking.
- o Pollution.
- o Fried and burnt foods.
- o Processed foods.
- o Drugs.
- o Alcohol.
- o UV radiation.
- o Stress.
- o Aging.
- o Exercise.

CREATE A FERTILE LIFE

We need a team of antioxidants for healthy functioning and optimal fertility, so this is why eating a diet rich in the antioxidant foods is so important. These main antioxidants are vitamins A, C, and E, selenium, coenzyme Q10, betacarotene, lipoic acid and zinc. Foods rich in antioxidants also tend to be deeply coloured: orange, purple, green, red, pink and yellow. So that is why a rainbow of vegetables on your plate with deep, rich colours and strong flavours are so important.

> **Seasonal eating tip:**
>
> Eat raw or lightly steam these antioxidant rich foods in the warm weather to retain their nutrients. Steam or cook into soups or stews rather than eating them raw in the cold weather to support healthy digestion and metabolism.

## 2. EAT TWO PIECES OF FRUIT PER DAY

Fruits are a great source of some of those essential fertility nutrients. Let's look at one of your fertility superfoods – blueberries. Packed full of antioxidants, blueberries are low in sugar so are a low-GI fruit, great for women with PCOS or people trying to lose weight. They are a good source of fibre, vitamin C, manganese and vitamin K. Best of all, they taste delicious! Be careful to choose organic berries as they are commonly sprayed (bugs really like berries too!). And look for local berries, as many berries available in major supermarkets have been shipped from across the globe, often China, which makes it harder to ensure the freshness and quality of your final product. Outside of summer, you might find it cheaper to buy frozen organic berries in bulk from the health food store. Of course there are plenty of fruits to choose from and we always encourage you to mix it up as much as possible - don't get stuck on a favorite! Variety is always the key. Mix it up as much as you can.

**Did you know that your intake of fruit and vegetables can improve your fertility?**

Following a Mediterranean diet, which includes a higher intake of fruits, vegetables and fish is associated with fewer couples consulting a physician for difficulties conceiving.[155]

A recent study found that the embryo quality of couples undergoing IVF was positively influenced by the consumption of fruit and vegetables in the diet.[156]

A further study of 161 couples doing IVF in the Netherlands found a preconception 'Mediterranean' diet (rich in fruit, vegetables and whole foods) contributed to the success of achieving pregnancy.[152]

## 3. DRINK 1.5–3 LITRES OF WATER A DAY (PREFERABLY FILTERED)

The uptake of nutrients into your body's cells is less than optimal if your cell's hydration is not ideal. All of our recommendations for your success depend on good hydration so this is an important focus. For more information on why filtered water is recommended; see Chapter 7 in the 10-step guide to a more fertility friendly environment.

## 4. EAT A HANDFUL OF MIXED SEEDS AND NUTS EVERY DAY

Nuts and seeds are little powerhouses of nutrients and they are even more nutrient-dense when eaten soaked, sprouted or activated. For example:

o Pumpkin seeds are a great source of zinc, one of the most important minerals for the growth and development of both sperm and eggs.

- Brazil nuts are a great source of the antioxidant selenium, which again is important for both sperm and egg quality. 3-4/day will give you a good dose of this important nutrient.

- Chia is another great fertility food, containing B vitamins, essential fatty acids, calcium, iron, and magnesium. Best of all, chia seeds are a complete vegetarian protein source containing all nine essential amino acids. Chia is also gluten-free and high in fibre. It absorbs water and forms a gelatinous texture, which is very soothing to our digestive tract, and great to get sluggish bowels moving!

- Quinoa is a gluten-free seed that can be cooked like a grain. It has less carbs and calories compared to white rice, and twice the protein – another of the few plant foods that contain all nine essential amino acids. It is also high in fiber, magnesium, B vitamins, iron, potassium, calcium, phosphorus, vitamin E and various beneficial antioxidants.

## How do I eat seeds?

Seeds are a great snack on their own or along with a piece of fruit, they can be dry roasted on low heat in the oven flavoured with a bit of tamari or sea salt, and they are great added to salads and stir fries.

Seeds can be ground (along with nuts) to make a mixture that is excellent when added to smoothies, porridge or yoghurt. Keep this stored in the freezer to keep the oils fresh if you grind more than you need at a time.

If you can, try to soak your seeds (and nuts for the same reason) for a few hours or overnight before eating. It will start to germinate, be easier to digest and contain more nutrients than an un-soaked seed. Dehydrate in the sun or low temp oven fully before storing again or eat immediately.

Add extra seeds to your muesli or toast in the morning.

Make a 'chia pudding' by combining one cup of coconut or almond milk with a quarter of a cup of chia seeds and one teaspoon of raw cacao. Leave to set in a jar, shaking a few times. Add a hand full of organic berries or soaked nuts or seeds and you have yourself an excellent quick breakfast or afternoon snack.

Look up a recipe for quinoa porridge or mix some cooked quinoa into your oat porridge to boost the protein content of your breakfast. Serve with extra soaked seeds, berries and yoghurt.

# 5. EAT FISH TWO TO THREE TIMES PER WEEK

Fish are a great source of both protein and omega 3 fats. Protein is essential for our growth, maintenance and repair of tissues, energy, the production of enzymes, blood cells and hormones, immune function and most importantly, reproductive function in both men and women.

As an added benefit to boosting your fertility by improving your protein intake, you'll also experience the other benefits of having adequate protein: improved hair, skin and nails, better mood and energy, improved muscle tone and strength, enhanced immunity and, if necessary, weight loss and appetite management... just to name a few! What a great list of side-effects!

Omega 3 fats are vital for hormonal balance and for sperm development, enhancing both sperm quality and morphology (shape) plus a healthy outer layer for the egg. Apart from fish, other sources of omega 3 fatty acids are flax seeds, hemp seeds, olive oil and nuts and seeds.

Of course, fresh is best but if tinned is your only option then choose tinned sardines or wild (not farmed) salmon. Unfortunately, these have their own drawback with the inner plastic lining often containing BPAs so try to limit these to just occasionally. See Chapter 7 the 10-step guide to a more fertility friendly environment for more information on this.

## Fish: A case of bigger not being better

Be careful to avoid the larger fish, which are more likely to be high in mercury. This heavy metal has the ability to cross the placenta and the blood-brain barrier and is definitely not healthy for us or our offspring! Deep sea, ocean, cold water fish are the ones with high omega 3 fats. Check that your fish is locally caught, or if from overseas ensure it's from clean waters (northern Europe, New Zealand). Avoid farmed and wild-caught fish from Asian regions, including prawns and shellfish.

| ✓ EAT THIS | ✗ NOT THIS* |
| --- | --- |
| Herring | Tuna |
| Mackerel | Shark/Flake |
| Mullet | Swordfish |
| Salmon | Barramundi |
| Sardines | King mackerel |
| Ocean trout | Shellfish |
| Pilchards | Orange Roughy (Deep Sea Perch) |
| Blue grenadier | Catfish |
| King George whiting | |

* Avoid or eat no more than once per month.

# 6. EAT PROTEIN-RICH FOODS AT MOST OF YOUR MEALS (YES THAT MEANS BREAKFAST, LUNCH AND DINNER)

Protein is not high on the radar for many people. This is probably at least partially due to the high availability and reliance on cheap, processed carbohydrates in our culture, which are very addictive and cause cravings. There's also a lack of understanding of the benefits of quality proteins in the diet. We are in no way recommending that you go out there and eat meat at every meal, however. While many fad weight loss diets of recent years can take the need for protein a little far, we do recommend learning about the importance of protein-rich foods, and that you eat as wide a variety of proteins as possible. This can be easier for meat and dairy eaters, but often they may be limiting their sources. For vegetarians and vegans, extra effort may be needed, but it is still very achievable and well worth your attention.

## Why is protein so important?

Amino acids found in proteins are the building blocks for our DNA and almost all our biological processes. Just to name a few:

o Reproductive function in both men and women.

o Growth, maintenance and tissue repair.

o Energy production.

o Blood cell and hormone production.

o Immune function.

o Hair, skin and nails.

o Muscle tone and strength.

o Mood and energy.

It is important to eat protein from varied sources, and not to eat too much protein of any one type. This particularly applies to meat and dairy, both of which may cause other health issues if eaten too often. It helps to complement your protein intake with plant-based sources such as nuts and legumes. See the table below for a rough guide to the number of ideal serves-per-week. If you can, choose free-range, organic and grass-fed dairy and red meats, which are much healthier protein choices than their grain-fed alternatives.

## Foods high in protein

| FOODS | IDEAL SERVES PER WEEK (SERVES = 150G) |
|---|---|
| Good quality red meat:<br>o Kangaroo.<br>o Organic and/or grass-fed lean beef.<br>o Organic lamb. | Two to four. |
| Organic chicken. | Two to four. |
| Fish. | Two to four. |
| Soy beans, edamame, tofu, tempeh and miso (eat traditional forms of organic soy, ensuring you avoid processed soy products and those containing 'soy protein isolate'). | Two to seven. |
| Legumes — lentils, beans, chickpeas and beans. | Two to seven. |
| Nuts and seeds, including nut butters, tahini etc. (Especially walnuts, almonds, brazil nuts, quinoa and seseme, pumpkin, chia and sunflower seeds). | A small handful daily. |

| | |
|---|---|
| Organic dairy, including sheep and goats milk products (yoghurt, quark, ricotta, feta, cheese). | Two to seven. |
| Organic eggs. | Two to seven (two eggs per serve). |

## How much protein do I need for optimal fertility?

As a general rule, you want to eat about one gram of protein per kilogram of body weight each day. An easy guide to help you to achieve this is to eat a palm-sized portion of protein at each meal (double this size for legumes and soy-based proteins), with some small added snacks in the form of nuts, seeds, dairy or eggs. Your protein requirements will also depend on varying factors such as your body weight and level of exercise.

## Protein for vegetarians

Vegetarians obviously don't eat meat (although some choose to eat fish), whilst others choose not to eat any food derived from an animal source (vegans). All plant foods have varying amounts of protein, but if you are getting most of your nutrition from plant-based sources you need to make sure you know about 'protein combining'.

The body makes proteins out of building blocks called amino acids. While animal sources of protein contain all the essential amino acids we require, plant-based proteins, other than soy, chia and quinoa, don't contain the full amino acid profile necessary for the body to make proteins. By combining your plant-based foods with other foods that contain more of the amino acid that is low or missing, you can achieve the full amino acid profile necessary for your fertility, good health and vitality.

The following combinations contain your full amino acid requirements:

o   Legumes combined with grains.

o   Legumes combined with nuts/seeds.

For example, dahl with rice, a salad with chickpeas and sunflower seeds, or baked beans on wholemeal toast will all give you your full amino acid requirements. Think of traditional food combinations from countries that rely on legumes and beans for their meals, and intuitively they will most likely have it right!

However, while the belief was that every amino acid needed to be supplied at the same meal, it's now thought that your body will store up the amino acids to make complete proteins from all the food you eat over the course of a day or so. As always, variety is the key! If you eat different combinations of grains, legumes, nuts, seeds, vegetables and fruits throughout the day, your protein requirements should be met.

And by variation, we mean really mix it up! Get out of your cooking rut and experiment with different foods. Vary the types of grains/legumes/ nuts/veggies. Many people rely on toast for breakfast, a sandwich for lunch and some bread or pasta for dinner! There are so many different choices available to you that will mean you get a much wider variety of nutrients available to support your health and fertility. And that's just grains!

## The soy question

Soy has many benefits. In its natural form, it is a complete protein and contains phytoestrogens and good amounts of vitamins and minerals such as B vitamins, magnesium, iron, folate, lecithin and calcium to name a few. But there does seem to be some mixed messages circulating about soy, and if you scratch the surface there is quite a fuss being made of this humble little bean. So, what is all the fuss about?

Traditionally, soy has been considered a staple of many Asian diets, generally only eaten as the cooked young bean (edamame) or as tofu or fermented products such as tamari, miso and tempeh. The low rates of menopause symptoms and some common cancers such as breast cancer in Asian (especially Japanese) communities have regularly been cited as good reasons to consume soy in our modern Western diet.

While the benefits seem clearer for our Asian neighbours, the soy topic has become hotly debated for us Westerners who have turned it into a highly-refined commercial product. Isolated soy extracts have become a low fat, low carb and low nutrient 'filler' or 'bulking agent' in many processed commercial products. Due to our love of these products, soy — once relegated to the realm of vegetarians and more 'alternative' types — has become a commonplace ingredient in our modern diet. In fact, the Australian Food and Grocery Council has found that about 50% of processed foods contain soy – it is in everything from bread, cereal, milk, 'healthy' frozen meals, pizzas and meat pies to baby formula, chewing gum, chocolate and margarine.

But according to some current research women trying to conceive are encouraged to eat soy to improve fertility.[157]

## So, is there a problem with soy?

The issues are both with the way we grow and process the soy, along with the way we consume it. Leaving the genetically-modified growing techniques aside (yes, much of our soy is GMO), soy is processed to extract the protein and leave the fat and carbohydrate component behind (and the nutrients!). You will find soy on the processed food labels as Textured Vegetable Protein (TVP), Textured Plant Protein (TPP), soy isoflavones or soy isolates. Our Asian friends — who seem to benefit from soy — are not known to pour it over their processed cereal or consume a ½ litre of soymilk in a protein shake rich with soy isolates. Further, some genetic studies show that those of Asian descent may have a genetic predisposition to metabolising the components of soy in a different and more beneficial way.[158]

A body of evidence suggests a worrying link between high soy intake and soy isolate consumption and infertility for both men and women.[159] Because it is in so many processed foods (even seemingly healthy processed foods), many people don't realise how much soy they are eating. Soy also contains goitrogens: substances that may suppress your thyroid function and can further contribute to fertility issues.

## So, should you eat soy?

| √ RECOMMENDED | X AVOID |
| --- | --- |
| Organic, whole soy bean products;<br>o  Tamari.<br>o  Miso.<br>o  Tempeh.<br>o  Natto.<br>o  Tofu.<br>o  Organic whole bean soymilk is fine, but as with all milk, mix it up. Try milk made from almonds, hazelnuts, quinoa, rice and even cows! | Processed soy;<br>o  Soy protein isolate.<br>o  TVP.<br>o  GMO soy (if the label doesn't say organic, it is likely to be GMO.<br>o  Soy junk foods (like soy cheese, vegetarian sausages or burgers and soy ice-cream).<br>o  Hydrogenated soybean oil.<br>o  Soy based protein powder.<br>o  Soy baby formula. |
| **How often?** There is much research to suggest one serve/day of soy is very good for your hormonal and overall health. This equals 100g tofu or 1 cup soy milk. We suggest eating it two to seven times a week. | If you are worried about your thyroid function, or you know you have an under active thyroid, it may be best to avoid soy. Individual advice is required here so check with your expert health practitioner. |

## IVF and protein

What were you planning for dinner? If your meals are high in carbohydrates and low in protein, your embryo quality may suffer. Women doing IVF who eat high levels of protein and low levels of carbohydrates had better quality eggs and embryos according to recent research.[159] Patients who switched to a low-carbohydrate, high-protein diet and then underwent another cycle increased their blastocyst formation rate from 19% to 45%, and their clinical pregnancy rate from 17% to 83%. For a positive effect on your fertility, a healthy weight is important, and the research recommends (on balance across the day) that you eat more than 25% protein and less than 40% carbs from your overall caloric intake.

# 7. SWAP WHITE ('REFINED') GRAINS FOR WHOLE-GRAINS

Unprocessed brown rice, oats, barley, rye, spelt, wheat, buckwheat, bulgar, millet, corn, quinoa, wholegrain breads (choose quality wholegrain sourdough, sprouted or paleo breads) and pastas (made from the whole-wheat grain) are all considered whole-grains. These are far better for your fertility (as well as your pregnancy outcomes once you have conceived) due to their nutrient density.

Compared with processed or refined grains like white rice, white bread and white flour (milled to remove the bran and germ for a finer texture and longer shelf-life), wholegrains are considered complex carbohydrates. They are more slowly absorbed into the blood stream, and don't cause such dramatic spikes in your blood-sugar levels (see below). Whole-grains contain significantly higher levels of fertility nutrients such as B vitamins, zinc, selenium and magnesium, as these are lost or destroyed in the processing to become refined products. They also include fibre, which of course is important for your digestive health, and interestingly, choosing whole-grains over refined grains has been linked to lower risks of heart disease, type 2 diabetes, cancer and more.

**Note:** wholegrain pastas are still made from whole-wheat that has been pulverised, diminishing many of the beneficial effects. Nonetheless, if you choose to eat pasta on the odd occasion, it is better to choose whole-grain pasta as it does contain more fibre and will tend to be more filling, contain fewer calories and more nutrients than refined pasta. Perhaps instead, try substituting your regular pasta dishes with a gluten-free whole-grain pasta like buckwheat or legume-based pasta. Even better, skip the pasta altogether and use beans, broccolini or thin peels of zucchini (use your peeler or try a spiraliser) as the base for your pasta sauce.

One very healthy wholegrain bread is Ezekiel bread, which you can generally find in the fridge at your health food store along with other sprouted bread varieties. It is made from a variety of whole-grains such as wheat, millet, barley and spelt as well as legumes. The grains and legumes in this bread are sprouted before they are cooked, increasing their nutrient content significantly. It is a rich, delicious and super satisfying bread experience! Try it with sliced tomatoes and hummus or toast it and add organic butter, sardines and a little sea salt. Yum!

### What's all the fuss about blood-sugars and what does it have to do with carbohydrates?

These days the negative effects of fluctuating blood-sugar levels are well recognised. When you consume sugar or a processed/refined carbohydrate (white flour products such as white bread and white rice, etc.), the simple molecules are quickly absorbed through the intestinal wall and enter your blood stream rapidly. This causes a spike in your blood-sugar levels, and as a response your body must quickly produce lots of insulin to get the levels down again.

The simplest way to explain this process is to compare it to a roller-coaster. When you eat processed carbs or sugars, your blood-sugar increases rapidly and you become what we call 'hyper glycaemic' (high blood-glucose). The responding insulin rush dramatically brings your blood-sugar levels down again, and you then crash and become 'hypo glycaemic' (low blood-glucose). When your blood-sugar is low you may feel tired, vague, sad, angry and hungry – a pretty unpleasant feeling we like to call 'hangry'! As your brain uses more glucose than any other organ in your body, it will direct you to seek out foods that will quickly increase your blood-sugar levels again – sugar and carbs. And then the roller-coaster starts all over again.

o  Do you crave high-carbohydrate foods?

o  Do you have a sweet tooth?

o  Or, are your cravings 'savoury' and you prefer to binge on chips, bread or pasta?

This really is a pre-diabetic pattern and if it isn't stopped, you increase your odds to develop Type 2 diabetes in the long run and fertility problems in the meantime.

Your liver also converts some of the glucose molecules into fats, leading to high cholesterol, 'fatty liver' and weight gain. We used to believe that high cholesterol was only caused by people eating a lot of fat, but it is now clear that having high blood-sugar can also lead to high cholesterol and can damage your blood vessels.

These high blood levels of glucose, insulin and fats are all heavily associated with poor fertility outcomes in men and women. Men are more likely to have poor sperm quality when they eat a lot of processed, sugary foods and women can develop ovulation issues as a result of these types of eating patterns.

An effective way to positively influence your blood-glucose levels is to always choose whole-grains (see above) and consume these complex carbs with some protein. The protein acts to slow the spike of blood-glucose, and helps to maintain adequate blood-sugar levels for longer, meaning that you are sustained for longer periods of time and will avoid the roller-coaster pattern.

For example, for breakfast you might have some eggs or sardines on wholemeal or sprouted toast, or muesli with natural yoghurt and nuts. You could choose a salad with salmon, a chicken sandwich on whole-grain bread or soup with chickpeas for lunch. You may then have fish and salad, meat and vegetables or a tofu stir fry with brown rice for dinner. All healthy options containing quality proteins that will help to support good blood-sugar balance.

## As a rule avoid sugar in all forms

Avoid all sweet things especially sugar, artificial sugar substitutes, cordial, soft drinks, fruit juices, cakes, lollies, chocolates and biscuits. Organic honey, real maple syrup and dried fruits can be used sparingly and not every day. Stevia can be used instead of artificial sweeteners. But do try to minimise all added sweet and sweetening extras wherever possible.

## What about low-carb diets?

Low-carb diets can be an effective way to lose weight and successfully manage blood-sugar levels, but they're not for everyone. Some people do very well not consuming many carbs, and mostly living on proteins and vegetables. Others just don't seem to be able to cope and have a drop in energy levels and mood. Don't beat yourself up if you can't achieve a low-carb diet – it's actually not necessary for health and it doesn't mean you can't lose weight if you need to. Just ensure you have your proteins at each meal and combine them with only complex carbohydrates. This way you will still achieve a healthy blood-sugar balance. As long as you're not eating too much food, getting a good balance and doing your exercise, you'll still lose weight.

# 8. EAT 'GOOD' FATS EVERY DAY

Essential fats are really important for our reproductive health. They are required for hormonal balance and thus impact ovulation and healthy egg function. They even have a role in reducing miscarriage risk. In pregnancy they may assist good blood flow to the uterus, reduce the risk of pre-eclampsia, pre-term birth, low weight baby and post-natal depression and are crucial for your baby's brain and neurological development.[160,161] For men these essential fats are equally important as they help good sperm shape and assist the sperm entering the egg.[162] In IVF, good essential fatty acids are also indicated so that our eggs and sperm are protected when they are frozen in some IVF techniques.[163]

Apart from our cellular health, fats are needed so that we can absorb essential fat-soluble vitamins like vitamin A, D, E and K. These vitamins are critical for our reproductive function, and intake of these is often lacking.

Two of the main groups of fats are omega 6 polyunsaturated fats and omega 3 fatty acids. A diet that is supportive of optimal fertility would include more omega 3 fatty acids and less omega 6 fatty acids.

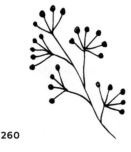

# The signs and symptoms of essential fatty acid deficiency

If you are overly deficient in essential fats you may see one or more of the following signs and symptoms:

### FERTILITY

Lack of ovulation or erratic menstrual cycle.

Dry vagina/inadequate fertile mucus production.

Abnormal sperm morphology.

Pre-menstrual symptoms.

Breast pain/tenderness.

### GENERAL HEALTH

Dry skin and lips.

Poor wound health and increased susceptibility to infection.

Fatigue, foggy thinking, poor memory.

Poor circulation.

Dandruff or dry hair.

Mood swings/depression.

Arthritis.

## Saturated and trans-fats

These have been linked to poor fertility and numerous chronic diseases. When consumed in high quantities they can become inflammatory in the body and cause cellular structures to be more rigid. In small amounts, saturated fats have good uses and we need saturated fats and cholesterol to make our reproductive hormones.

When oils are exposed to sunlight or excessive heat, or have become old, their structure changes (they turn rancid) and can be more harmful than good. So buy small amounts of fresh nuts and oils regularly rather than buying in bulk and consider keeping them in the fridge.

| BETTER FATS TO EAT (ORGANIC WHERE POSSIBLE) | MINIMISE YOUR INTAKE OF THE FOLLOWING |
| --- | --- |
| Cold pressed oils e.g. extra virgin olive oil, macadamia nut or flaxseed oil. | Baked goods e.g. cakes, biscuits. |
| Avocado. | Highly processed and fast foods. |
| Oily fish like salmon and sardines. | Fried foods. |
| Seeds e.g. pumpkin, sesame, sunflower, chia, linseeds, quinoa. | Margarine, olive oil spreads. |
| Nuts e.g. brazil, walnuts, almonds etc. | Vegetable oils, "light" olive oil. |
| Small amounts of butter (1-2 tsp/day). | Avoid low-fat products e.g. low-fat milk. |
| For cooking; coconut, macadamia, olive oil, butter or ghee. | |

## No, no, no – please do not eat low-fat dairy.

Check out the ingredients on the low-fat products and most likely they will be high in sugar. Sugar is one of the things we want to avoid for weight and blood-sugar management, fertility, and overall health. Not only that but having low-fat dairy products may actually be hazardous for fertility. A Harvard study analysed data of 18,555 women from the Nurses Health Study II and concluded that women consuming full-fat milk and dairy products had a better chance of conceiving, while eating low-fat dairy could hamper fertility and affect ovulation.[106]

## What oils should we cook with?

Keep your olive oil and other oils in a dark glass container away from direct sunlight. As a general rule, we don't recommend deep frying or cooking in high temperatures but if you are going to fry then use small amounts of one of the more stable saturated fats like coconut, butter, or ghee. Olive oil with its higher monounsaturated content is a good choice for low temperature frying. We suggest using a good quality, cold-pressed, extra virgin olive oil — when lightly frying, reduce the heat damage by adding the food to the fry pan before the oil heats up or add a little water to keep the temperature down.

## Are margarines, olive spread and other spreads better for my health than butter?

In order for any vegetable oils to be made solid they have to be heated to a very high temperature and have hydrogen pumped through them to make them solidify. This hydrogenation makes them act like a saturated fat in the body, and margarines can have up to 40% of trans-fats. Now we know trans-fats are not good for our arteries and general health. The upshot of all this is that our body has a difficult time in getting rid of these processed fats and can't utilise them very well. So, although butter is a saturated fat and we don't want too much of that, it does have the advantage of not being highly processed and being full of those great fat-soluble vitamins A, D and E plus some minerals like calcium, magnesium and potassium. So please do have butter but use sparingly and always choose organic (one to two teaspoons a day is definitely good for us) or put olive oil or avocado on your bread instead.

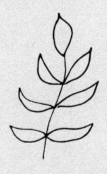

# TOP TIPS FOR HIM AND HER

Stretch your imagination and scope for eating a truly broad and colourful diet rich with variety.

Eat the recommended intake of five serves (approximately three cups) of vegetables a day and make sure it's a rainbow of colours. That means thinking up creative ways of getting colour into breakfast, lunch and dinner, which actually isn't that hard: think blueberries and strawberries with breakfast, a salad of greens, beetroot, capsicum and squash with lunch and a stir fry of chick peas, cauliflower, broccoli, corn, carrots and fresh herbs with your choice of protein for dinner.

The Mediterranean diet rich in fruit and vegetables has been shown to be a winner for fertility

Drink 1.5-3 litres of filtered water daily to ensure uptake of nutrients into your cells and to keep hydrated.

Eat a handful of raw, unsalted nuts and seeds everyday.

Eat fish 2-3 times a week and choose the smaller fish like sardines, herring, salmon or ocean trout. Be careful to avoid the larger fish, which are more likely to be high in mercury. This heavy metal has the ability to cross the placenta and the blood-brain barrier and are definitely not healthy for us or our offspring!

Eat some protein at each of your three main meals.
Essential for reproductive function in both men and women.

Eating quality, organic, whole bean soy products
is fine for fertility and may even be beneficial.
Aim for two to seven times a week.

Blood-sugar balance is a cornerstone of good health
including fertility health. Avoid all sweet things especially
sugar, artificial sugar substitutes, cordial, soft drinks, fruit
juices, cakes, lollies and biscuits. Organic honey, real maple
syrup and dried fruits can be used sparingly.

Swap white refined grains like white bread, pasta and rice
for wholegrains. Healthy blood-sugar balancing grains
are those that you would consider to be wholegrain.
Unprocessed brown rice, oats, barley, rye, spelt, wheat,
buckwheat, bulgar, millet, corn, quinoa, wholegrain
breads and pastas are all considered wholegrains.
These are far better for your fertility as well as your
pregnancy outcomes once you have conceived.

Eat your 'good' fats daily for hormonal balance
and healthy ovulation and egg and sperm function.

# TOP TIPS FOR HIM AND HER

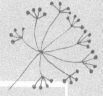

Choose full-fat dairy as low-fat dairy has been
linked with fertility issues.

Cook with fats like coconut, butter, or ghee for
high temperature cooking. Olive oil with its higher
monounsaturated content is a good choice for low
temperature frying and better consumed cold or added at
the end of cooking. We suggest using a good quality,
cold-pressed, extra virgin olive oil.

Avoid margarines, olive and vegetable oil spreads,
instead use olive oil, avocado, nut butters or a small
amount of butter.

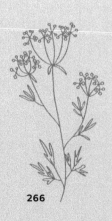

CREATE A FERTILE LIFE

# 10

# Six more steps and superfoods for fertility

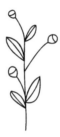

**I already eat a healthy diet and follow the top eight daily; what else can I do with my diet to improve my fertility?**

Once you have the top eight covered then as the icing on the cake (so to speak! Of course we won't be suggesting cake or icing!) you can enhance your fertility even further by incorporating the following six suggestions as much as possible too.

## 1. WE RECOMMEND EATING LOCALLY AND IN SEASON WHERE POSSIBLE

Eating a seasonal diet ensures the foods you do consume are as fresh as possible and are consumed when they are picked – not after they have been stored for a year or two. Did you know that an apple you purchase from the supermarket may have been in storage for up to two years before it reached the supermarket shelf?

Very few foods are readily available all year round, and yet, if you shop exclusively in supermarkets you could be forgiven for thinking that tomatoes and zucchini, mangoes and bananas grow everywhere all year 'round. Actually, most products have been in storage, often with special coatings of wax or plastic or artificially gas-ripened to enable them to survive travelling sometimes thousands of miles only to be stored for long periods of time before they hit the supermarket shelf. Special coatings, refrigeration and other technologies can keep food for much longer than nature intended. Though they still look ok, non-organic, long-stored food loses nutrients and quality the longer it sits on the shelf, meaning you are getting a lesser quality item on your plate! Of course, it is cheaper (saying nothing about the paltry amounts the grower receives), you are paying for less.

Seek out your local farmers or other market to purchase the bulk of your fresh food items (many growers in these contexts use chemical-free growing techniques though they may not be certified organic). The feeling of handing your hard-earned cash to the person who put the hard work into growing your food is a uniquely heartening experience. Hearing them say "I picked these yesterday" is confirmation of the incredible freshness and quality of the product you are purchasing. If it costs a little more, remember your money goes back into your local community, directly to the grower and you are buying a higher quality, more nutritious product.

Your local health food store is your next best bet for fresh food and also will make it easier to buy fresh, seasonal produce.

CREATE A FERTILE LIFE

# 2. CHOOSE ORGANIC FOODS

There are many excellent reasons to consider making the change to including as much organic produce in your diet as possible. Here are a few that we find compelling:

## Pesticides and other chemicals have not been proven safe

Most pesticides and other chemicals used in agriculture have a detrimental effect on the nervous or reproductive systems of life forms considered to be pests. Importantly, while individual chemicals may seem ok, there is little evidence to prove the safety of these chemicals once they start mixing together – either in our bodies, through multiple applications of different chemical compounds in the same context, or through accumulation in the environment (soils, rivers, oceans, our bodies, food and the air). The cumulative effect of repeated ingestion along with the combined effect of multiple chemicals acting together are poorly understood, researched and tested. To fully research, with so many chemicals in popular use, would be incredibly time consuming, complex and difficult. We prefer to err on the side of caution and go with what is proven – chemical free!

### How do I know it is really organic?

In Australia there are a number of organisations that provide an 'official' certified organic stamp (meaning it is actually organic food). All these organisations, such as National Association for Sustainable Agriculture Australia (NASAA), Australian Certified Organic (ACO) must comply with the Australian National Standards. There are currently only seven certified organisations, so look for their stamp when purchasing organic food. Some farmers grow without chemicals but are not certified organic and you will find them through your local farmers markets and local green grocers.

## Organic tastes better and has been shown to have higher nutrient values than conventionally grown food

This is particularly true of conventional food that has been stored or otherwise treated to preserve longevity. The longer it takes from the time your food is picked to the time you consume it, the more that happens to that food between picking and eating, the more compromised its nutrition, longevity and most importantly, its taste! Many foods are developed with storage and transportation over taste as primary considerations. The proof really is in the tasting.

There is research reinforcing both sides of the nutrition question when it comes to comparing organic and produce grown using chemicals. We consider this a moot point since organic trumps chemically grown every time when it comes to taste and the unwelcome effects of pesticides.

## Something to consider... Is cheap food really better?

Why do we expect food to be cheap anyway? This is a really interesting question. It seems many people want multiple flat screen TVs and many other luxuries in their homes they are willing to pay considerable sums for, yet when it comes to food, they expect to get it at rock-bottom prices. When you consider the importance of food in maintaining wellness, this seems crazy. As we have already discussed there are a number of reasons why cheap food is undesirable, unethical and less good for you. It is simply a matter of shifting priorities and making choices that support and enhance your well-being.

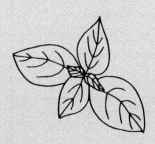

     CREATE A FERTILE LIFE

## If cost really is your motivator, grow your own

Of course, growing your own is the best way to know where your food has come from and what is on it. Start with something simple like fresh herbs, lettuces and other greens. These are quick growing and a good way to build your confidence in the garden. Even those with only a small space can achieve quite a lot and there are loads of books on the market showing you how to make the most of whatever space you have available. If you have a back yard, few things are more satisfying than keeping chooks for the healthiest eggs around. Chickens are a surprisingly low-maintenance, low-cost pet, and will demolish your kitchen scraps, provide valuable manure for your garden and will eat whatever garden bugs and pests they can find.

## I can't afford to eat all my food organic. Which foods are essential to have organic?

A great general rule is that whatever we know bugs love to eat are the things that are most commonly and problematically sprayed with pesticides. Things that have their own thick skin or are grown underground have a little more protection from direct spraying (think avocados and onions). Use the following 'Dirty Dozen™' as a guide to what you should absolutely buy organically if you can, and the things you can afford to compromise on. For more information check out the 'Shoppers Guide to Pesticides in Produce™' by the Environmental Working Group at *www.ewg.org*. These lists are updated as of 2019.

### DIRTY DOZEN ™

| | | |
|---|---|---|
| 1. Strawberries | 5. Apples | 9. Pears |
| 2. Spinach | 6. Grapes | 10. Tomatoes |
| 3. Kale | 7. Peaches | 11. Celery |
| 4. Nectarines | 8. Cherries | 12. Potatoes |

| | | |
|---|---|---|
| 1. Avocadoes | 6. Papayas | 11. Cauliflower |
| 2. Sweet Corn | 7. Eggplants | 12. Cantaloupes |
| 3. Pineapples | 8. Asparagus | 13. Broccoli |
| 4. Sweet Peas (frozen) | 9. Kiwi Fruit | 14. Mushrooms |
| 5. Onions | 10. Cabbage | 15. Honeydew Melons |

**NB:** The Environmental Working Group are an American based organisation and they produce this list yearly. This list may not be 100% accurate for Australia, but we know of no comparable list here. This is still a good basic guide.

# 3. RAW VERSUS COOKED?

We often get asked this question and it really depends on the season, the climate, your circulation and the strength of your digestive function. As a rough guide, the warmer it is and the stronger your digestion and circulation, the more raw foods you can have. In winter, and especially if you feel the cold and often experience bloating or digestive issues, you will be much better with soups, stews and other warm, easy-to-digest foods. However, if you are in a hot climate and generally have a good digestion then more salads, sprouts and raw recipes will be fine for you.

## Chinese medicine and the importance of warm foods

Traditional Chinese medicine is all about maintaining homeostasis in the body. We understand pathology in the body by understanding what factors have thrown it out of balance: heat, cold, damp, etc. When we eat cold food, our core temperature drops, and our body must use energy to warm the food up to our internal body temperature. This enables adequate digestion and absorption, but it also unnecessarily uses a lot of energy. When we eat warm, neutral or balanced foods, our body doesn't have to expend so much energy preparing it for digestion and assimilation, so we use less overall energy. This means our body can put that energy to better use elsewhere – and eating is not using more energy than it should.

Particular organs also dislike certain conditions. For example, the spleen dislikes damp. When we eat too many cold foods, which can lead to damp, we might experience symptoms such as lethargy in general or, after eating, loose stools, bloating and undigested food in stools. Correcting your intake of cold foods will see a quick turn-around in symptoms. This is particularly important in cold climates and during winter.

## How do I know if food is balanced, neutral, warm or cold?

It is actually pretty simple:

All food has both a temperature (depending on whether it is refrigerated or cooked) as well as a thermal nature, which doesn't change. This means regardless of whether it is cooked or refrigerated, it is still warm or cold. For example, milk is considered cool and damp.

You can make it better by warming it up and adding warming things to balance it out. For example, Chai tea is full of warming spices (cinnamon, cardamom, ginger, etc. – not the powdered version some cafés serve, which is just flavoured sugar – the real tea made with whole spices), which can help to balance out the cold and damp quality of the milk.

Slow-cooked foods (energy in) are more warming than things that are eaten raw. Things grown in season are usually an appropriate food for that season – for example, root vegetables in winter – another good reason to eat seasonally! A good general rule is to try to not eat foods, such as fruit, straight out of the fridge and always have water at room temperature.

Pair cool or neutral foods with warming foods to create balance (for example: sushi (cool) with ginger (warm) or yogurt (cool) with baked apples and cinnamon (warm).

If you tend to feel the cold, a daily cup of ginger tea is beneficial. Simply put a couple of slices of raw ginger in either boiling water, or even black tea with milk.

## 4. PREPARED VERSUS PROCESSED

Preparing your own food means you know exactly what goes into it. Also, when we cook for ourselves we eat differently than when we dine out or eat take away food. This leads to higher consumption of foods that really take too much effort to eat regularly at home. Consider chips: scrub and peel your potatoes, cut them up, fry them in oil, drain them and after you've enjoyed them you need to figure out what to do with the oil. Eating out saves all this effort, so you indulge more often.

We eat more simply most of the time when we prepare food at home. You'll also save money as cooking at home is invariably cheaper than eating out and save on lunches by taking left-overs to work. It takes a little more organisation, but you'll eat far higher quality foods if you can make the time to prepare them yourself.

## 5. ADD IN SOME SUPER FERTILITY FOODS

There is a lot of talk about superfoods and all the amazing things they have to offer for just about every conceivable human ailment and worry. From cacao to maca to goji and acai the promises include increased fertility, cures for cancer, recovery from all sorts of disease, anxiety and woe. Certainly, these foods have so much to offer and can definitely be considered powerful, high-quality, nutrient-dense foods. Please don't be fooled into thinking these superfoods are the be all and end all.

Superfoods are a useful and highly beneficial addition to your diet. But no amount of goji berries is going to make up for a general diet of chips, soft drinks and take-away foods. Eating any kind of superfood does not equalise or diminish the effects of the two or three coffees or cokes you might drink in a day or if you gorge on junk food week after week. If you haven't got the basics covered, superfoods are not your miracle cure-all for a modern-day poor lifestyle.

In fact, you may be surprised by our list of superfoods – it is not all goji berries and expensive exotics like Acai powder. It's the bulk of our daily food intake that has the fertility boosting effect and superfoods are like adding in the frills.

## Here are our tips for the daily, essential top superfoods for fertility and health!

### GREEN LEAFY VEGETABLES

Include as many different greens on your plate every day. Variety is the key! While being a great source of fibre, they're packed full of folate and such a big variety of essential nutrients at the top of our healthy reproductive needs. Include silverbeet, spinach, rocket, kale, chard, all types of lettuce, parsley, coriander, dill, mint, etc.

### BLUEBERRIES

This antioxidant and phytonutrient rich, low-glycaemic index (low GI) super berry is full of nutrients and fibre. They are anti-inflammatory and antiaging, and perfect if you are trying to lose weight or improve your blood-sugar. Best of all, they taste delicious! Be careful to choose organic with all berries as they are commonly sprayed (bugs really like berries too!). Look for local berries as many berries available in major supermarkets have been shipped from across the globe, often China, which makes it harder to ensure the freshness and quality of your final product.

> **Sweet pudding recipe.**
>
> Quick, easy and super nutritious: stew rhubarb and apple with
> a handful of local or frozen organic blueberries thrown in at the
> end. Add a little water, lots of cinnamon (great for your blood-
> sugar and taste buds!) and a couple of spoons of chia seeds.
> Leave for ten minutes so the chia can absorb the water and
> become gelatinous, forming a lovely pudding-like texture

## EGGS

Free range, organic eggs are one of our best sources of protein,
vitamin D, B12, zinc, phosphorus and selenium. They are packed with
nutrients that are important from an egg and sperm-health point of
view. Yes, they contain cholesterol, so if it is a problem for you, take
fish oil at the same time to lessen the absorption of cholesterol. Also,
as part of a healthy diet that is low in saturated fat and high in healthy
fats, a little cholesterol is required. Cholesterol has been painted as
the bad guy, but it is also what our hormones are synthesized from.
If cholesterol is an issue, check with your naturopath about how to use
food to regain control!

## FERMENTED FOODS AND YOGHURT

Organic, full-fat, unflavoured, unsweetened yoghurt contains calcium,
good fats and 'friendly bacteria' to keep your digestive system healthy
and support optimal absorption of those all-important fertility
nutrients. Fermented foods such as sauerkraut, miso, tempeh and kefir
(as outlined in the next chapter all about digestion and fertility) are
also an important variety addition for the healthiest microbiome.

## QUINOA

While technically a seed, quinoa cooks up like a grain and unlike most
(even whole) grains, quinoa is a complete protein i.e. it contains all nine

essential amino acids. It also contains more fibre than other grains, and is rich in essential fatty acids, iron, lysine (great if you suffer from cold sores), magnesium, B2 and manganese. Quinoa is also gluten free. It is a significantly better grain choice than pasta or even brown rice due to its protein and nutrient content, and as we know how important good protein sources are for fertility then it is an excellent superfood to make friends with.

## SARDINES

This little fish is one of the richest sources of anti-inflammatory omega 3 fatty acids. They are also high in protein, zinc, and B vitamins, especially B6, folate and B12, vitamins A, D, E and K, which are vital nutrients for healthy hormone balance and reducing any inflammation in the body that may impact fertility. Eat them with the bones for the added bonus of calcium! Sardines are low on the food chain, so they are not high in mercury.

## OATS

High in soluble fibre, whole oats eaten daily have been shown to lower and help maintain healthy cholesterol and blood pressure. They improve bowel function and are a good source of B vitamins, vitamin E, magnesium, zinc and selenium – many of the best nutrients for fertility. Oats are also considered to be a 'nervine tonic' in herbal medicine, which means they are useful for calming and nourishing the nervous system. A steaming bowl of porridge topped with some of these other superfoods like chia seeds, walnuts, berries and yoghurt is a perfect breakfast. You can even try combining oats and quinoa for a porridge with a twist.

## WALNUTS

Researchers from UCLA in California found that men who ate a couple of handfuls of walnuts (75gms) a day saw improvements in their semen quality.[164] They found improvements in sperm motility and morphology. The suggestion is that it is because walnuts are a rich source of alpha-linolenic acid (an omega 3). Other benefits are brain and heart health with these great fats. Be sure the walnuts taste fresh and are organic.

## GOJI BERRIES

Goji Berries are one of the most commonly touted superfoods and are well regarded for their antioxidant properties. They have long been used in traditional Chinese medicine to nourish yin (blood and fluids in the body) and are also considered to be effective in managing diabetes and high blood pressure.

Goji berries contain many nutrients beneficial for fertility, including vitamins A, B and C, bioflavonoids, amino acids, and some essential fatty acids. These nutrients largely act as antioxidants, meaning that regular consumption of goji berries along with most other types of berries, can contribute to egg and sperm quality and assist in good endometrial development and blood flow to the uterus. The added benefit of low sugar levels and possible positive impact on blood-sugar levels further contribute to their reputation as a fertility superfood.

As with all berries, it is important to ensure you are consuming only organic goji's, especially as they are often grown in China where pesticide use is of specific concern.

## BEST EVER SUPERFOOD?

Anything you grow yourself. Nothing is more nutritious than something you have loved and tended in your own garden – pesticide-free and picked fresh to eat that day. There is NO better way to ensure freshness, ultimate nutrient content, maximum flavour and peak satisfaction and enjoyment.

# What about Maca?

This must be the most touted superfood ever on all the fertility blogs and web posts around. You'll find claims of its supersonic abilities to balance hormones, lift libido, boost energy, improve mood and enhance your fertility. Is this true? Well evidence to support these claims are limited, which isn't the same as saying it doesn't still have some therapeutic benefit. It certainly has many minerals, vitamins and protein and some studies show a benefit for men's sexual function, benefit for sperm production and improving progesterone levels and sex drive. This vegetable is traditionally eaten regularly in South America, and is thought to enhance fertility and treat menstrual disorders. To gain any potential benefits you would probably need to take Maca for at least 12 weeks on a therapeutic dose and there may be other better-studied herbs to choose instead.

# 6. SOAK, ACTIVATE, AND SPROUT!

Without going into too much detail, some foods are at their best when first soaked prior to cooking or eating. This applies to nuts, grains, seeds and legumes in particular. Soaking helps to reduce phytic acid, which in short can contribute to some of the digestive issues commonly associated with eating these foods (such as flatulence, bloating, digestive pain, etc.). Phytic acid appears to inhibit some enzyme activity and can also inhibit nutrient absorption, particularly minerals that are abundant in these foods.

To make life easy do a mass soak when you have time, so you always have soaked nuts, grains or legumes ready when you need them. One weekend you'll have bowls all over the kitchen for 24 hours but then you won't need to soak again for a little while. After soaking, simply drain and freeze portions for later use. This simple bit of organisation makes healthy eating so much easier.

Everything needs a different amount of soaking time. As a general rule, nuts and grains that you want to use for breakfast can just be soaked overnight: 8-12 hours will be plenty. For legumes and grains to have on hand, soak overnight, strain, refresh the water and soak again until the end of the day. Around 24 hours should see them just germinated and ready for cooking (or portioning up and freezing). If you want to go even further, you can soak your nuts then dehydrate them for optimum digestibility and nutritional excellence.

**Did you know that your freezer works optimally when full?**
If it is empty it is just keeping air cold which has no mass and so is harder to keep cold and stable. Filling your freezer with pre-prepared food items not only makes your life easier, but also makes your fridge more energy efficient! Who knew?

## Sprouting

Sprouted seeds, grains, nuts and legumes are not only more digestible, but being alive, they have substantially more nutrients and enzymes available than their unsprouted equivalent. They also don't require cooking, or need much less cooking. Each thing will take a different amount of time to sprout, but all you need to do after an initial overnight soak, is keep them moist by rinsing with water each day until you see a little green sprout emerge. This is one of those little things that can become a kitchen obsession and you'll find heaps of resources through your internet search engine.

# TOP TIPS FOR HIM AND HER

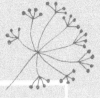

Eat locally and in season when available.

Eat organic foods - as much as possible.

As a rough guide, the warmer it is and the stronger
your digestion and circulation, the more raw foods
you can have. In winter, and especially if you feel
the cold and often experience bloating or digestive
issues, you will be much better with soups, stews
and other warm, easy-to-digest foods.

Aim to eat home prepared, quality food 90% of the time.

Superfoods are a useful and highly beneficial addition
to your diet. However if you haven't got the basics
covered, superfoods are not your miracle cure-all
for a modern-day poor lifestyle.

Our superfood list to include regularly in your daily foods:
green leafy veggies, blueberries, eggs, fermented foods,
quinoa, sardines, oats, walnuts and goji berries.

Grow your own veggies to secure the quality
of your veggies and to save money.

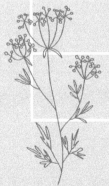

Learn how to soak, activate and sprout
your grains, seeds, nuts and legumes.

# 11

# Nutritional supplements for fertility

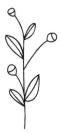

## CAN I DO ANYTHING ELSE TO ENHANCE MY FERTILITY NUTRITIONALLY? THE SUPPLEMENT QUESTION.

Supplementation is often essential to ensure a replete nutritional status. Many people are resistant to taking supplements believing that food alone should provide all that is required. There are a large number of compelling reasons why this is not necessarily the case. Many factors can result in less than optimal nutritional status even when you are following a good diet. These factors may include: stress, illness, poor digestion, food allergies/intolerances, coffee/tea/ alcohol, take-away food consumption, smoking, fad diets, medications (e.g. antibiotics, laxatives, contraception and anti-depressants can deplete various nutrients), lack of sunlight, shift workers, high exercise levels, long-term oral contraceptive use, past or current pregnancy and, of course, our own individual makeup and genetic factors (bio-individuality).

Even PMT may be an indicator of nutrient deficiency. Research has demonstrated that up to 60 per cent of women suffering from symptoms of premenstrual tension, such as headaches, irritability, bloating, breast tenderness, lethargy and depression can benefit from supplementation with vitamin B6.[165] Essential fatty acids and magnesium also have a role to play in overcoming PMT symptoms.[166,167] Past use of the oral contraceptive pill may have decreased absorption of folic acid and increased the need for vitamin B2, B6, B12 and vitamin C and E, zinc, magnesium and selenium.

## FOOD AS MEDICINE

Many people want their food to be their medicine but still do not eat anywhere near adequate amounts of nutrients required for food to function beyond mere sustenance. To treat disease, nutrients need to be taken in therapeutic doses to see benefit, under the care of an experienced practitioner. Lower doses do not have the same effect. The approach of your practitioner is very often going to be beyond the action of merely replacing nutrients not being obtained through diet; elevating food and nutrients to their highest potential in health and healing.

Cooking or reheating of meat and vegetables can oxidise and destroy heat susceptible vitamins. Food storage affects nutrients including long term refrigeration and freezing food. Transportation of food and length of time from picking to plate will deplete the nutrients. Many agricultural soils are deficient in trace elements – especially in Australia where topsoil levels are thin due to decades of intensive agriculture.

A diet overly dependent on highly-refined carbohydrates such as sugar, white flour and white rice, places greater demand on additional sources of B-group vitamins to process these carbohydrates. Convenience foods tend to be highly processed, often loaded with preservatives to improve shelf-life and tend to be overly reliant on poor quality fats or too much sugar to ensure flavour.

Even if you have cleaned up your diet recently, have you always been eating this way? Have there been periods in your life where you may have been depleted by less than healthy choices? Supplementation may be necessary for a while to correct any deficiencies or imbalances, and this is especially true if you are not in optimal health for any reason – fertility related or not.

## ARE THERE DANGERS TO SUPPLEMENTING?

Of course, high-dose nutrients and herbal supplements, like all medicines, absolutely must be taken only under the supervision of a qualified and experienced practitioner. There are dangers for even the most simple of nutrients. For example, if you have the genetic condition haemochromatosis, taking simple iron is extremely dangerous and can lead to organ damage. Many supplements will interfere with medications and some will compete for absorption with others. Taking high doses in one may deplete another, causing a different raft of complications. Caution is required.

Other nutrients are specifically harmful to an unborn baby during pregnancy at high doses such as iron, vitamin A and selenium, so self-prescribing nutrients for your fertility can be dangerous. Doses need to be carefully managed, reviewed and monitored over time with your health improvements and changing circumstances.

Nutritional medicine is a very safe and effective approach to improving a wide range of health conditions when supervised by an experienced practitioner such as a naturopath.

# A WORD OF WARNING ABOUT BUYING SUPPLEMENTS FROM OVERSEAS

Do you know that supplements purchased online from overseas may not contain what it says it does on the label, may contain the wrong ingredient or even be intentionally tainted with undeclared substances or other therapeutic agents?

In Australia, the TGA regulates manufacturers, ensuring quality. The manufacturing plants and laboratories are licenced and inspected to ensure they follow the highest standards and there are strict regulations about advertising claims too. Products purchased from overseas are not subject to the same high level of scrutiny.

Be very wary about making any online purchases, and only do so on the recommendation of a qualified healthcare professional or from a known and reputable source, and only if it fits your regime of other supplements too.

# WHAT SUPPLEMENTATION DO YOU NEED?

We are not in favour of blanket supplementation recommendations for all, although we do suggest a basic minimum of a comprehensive multivitamin and mineral formula (specific for male fertility, female preconception or pregnancy) and a good quality fish oil for both men and women for the three months before and during trying to conceive. Over and above this, each individual is different and needs to be prescribed a specific program of nutrient supplementation and herbal medicine regime to fit their picture. This is particularly true if IVF or other fertility drugs or hormones are being used. No two people are the same and we do not believe in a one-size-fits-all approach.

As stated above, while nutrients and herbal medicines provide a safe and effective approach to health care, they still carry risk and should not be toyed with lightly. We are not supporters of random acts of self-prescription and time and again have seen patients inappropriately self-prescribing nutrients and medicines based on something they have read in a book, on the Internet or on the recommendation of a well-meaning friend.

Fertility is an especially sensitive area. Playing with readily available herbal supplements that have hormonal implications can not only play havoc with your hormones but can be downright dangerous if you are undergoing IVF or other treatment.

## Folate and Vitamin D deserve a special mention

### Folate (folic acid) of course

Most of us are aware of the importance of folic acid when trying to conceive and often start a preconception multivitamin/mineral for that reason. Low levels of folic acid can increase the risk of neural tube issues such as spina bifida and supplementation has been shown to reduce this risk. Folate is important for egg and sperm development and as the neural tubes close over by week 8 of the pregnancy, it is advised to start on this nutrient prior to conception. Many of its important functions happen before you even know you are pregnant! Other vitamins like B12 and choline are also needed for neural tube development which is why a comprehensive fertility multivitamin is recommended. If you are able to consult a naturopath check which form of folate and dose is right for you.

Food sources: green leafy veggies (like kale, spinach, lettuce) beans and green beans, broccoli, peas, asparagus, Brussel sprouts, lentils, avocado.

## Vitamin D

We know of the important role vitamin D plays for our bone health and mood. It is also essential for fertility for making the hormone progesterone, stimulating follicles and egg maturation, and has a role in our reproductive organ function.[168] Optimal levels are likely to improve ovulation and reduce PMS. Vitamin D improves insulin sensitivity and low levels may be associated with impaired fertility, endometriosis, auto-immune conditions and PCOS. Low levels are associated with miscarriage, gestational diabetes, pre-eclampsia and low birth weight babies. In pregnancy it protects the baby against infection. Having good levels of vitamin D may also improve pregnancy success in IVF.

Deficiency is common, and research suggests 75% of Australian's are deficient so testing is recommended and adequate supplementation as needed.

Food sources: cod liver oil (stop when pregnant), oily fish (salmon, mackerel, sardines), eggs, liver (organic only).

Sunshine source: Levels needed will depend on skin pigment and dryness or any rashes like eczema. Approximately 15% of skin exposed to the sunshine for 10 minutes in summer and 20 minutes in winter between 11am-3pm daily will boost your vitamin D levels. Sunscreen will block vitamin D, however be careful not to burn.

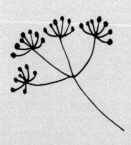

# DOSE

The complexity of these supplements requires an appropriate practitioner for both frequency and amount; drug/herb interactions; testing for need and repletion and monitoring implications of long-term use. We see many patients who have been taking a popular over-the-counter multivitamin for a very long time. Not only is the supplement not appropriate to their needs or not supplying adequate amounts of the right nutrients, there is also the issue that long-term use is not appropriate for many nutrients. Some nutrients can affect levels of other nutrients if taken for too long or at too high doses (case dependent) and many people lose the effectiveness of their multi-vitamin by taking an inappropriate multi or taking the same thing for years at a time.

Under the care of an appropriate practitioner you can safely and effectively manage your health and well-being. There is so much you can do to take control and contribute to your health regime and improved fertility with supportive diet and lifestyle change. This is where you need to take the reins. Let an expert take care of the tricky stuff!

# TOP TIPS FOR HIM AND HER

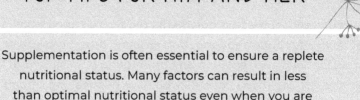

Supplementation is often essential to ensure a replete nutritional status. Many factors can result in less than optimal nutritional status even when you are following a good diet.

To treat a health issue, nutrients need to be taken in 'therapeutic doses' similar to pharmaceuticals under the care of an experienced practitioner. Lower doses do not have the same effect.

Change your diet if it's overly dependent on highly-refined carbohydrates such as sugar, white flour and white rice. There is greater demand on additional sources of B-group vitamins to process these carbohydrates.

High-dose nutrients and herbal supplements, like all medicines, absolutely must be taken only under the supervision of a qualified and experienced practitioner. There are dangers for even the most simple of nutrients. For example, if you have the genetic condition haemochromatosis, taking simple iron is extremely dangerous and can lead to organ damage.

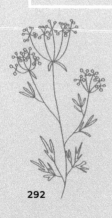

Don't buy your supplements from overseas as they may not contain what it says on the label, may contain the wrong ingredient or even be intentionally tainted with undeclared substances or other therapeutic agents.

As a basic minimum during the three months before conception and during pregnancy, ensure that you are taking a quality natal multivitamin with good folate levels and a quality fish oil.

Don't self-prescribe supplements as each individuals needs are different and a full assessment by a health professional is the safest approach.

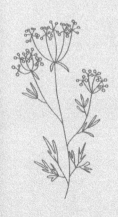

# 12

# Gut health, the microbiome and your fertility

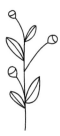

Naturopaths view digestion as the cornerstone for optimal functioning of the entire body. A poor-functioning digestive system can impact on all areas of our health, including mood, energy, immunity, skin and our fertility. Researchers agree that our gut, and specifically the billions of bacteria that reside there, are key to our health and fertility outcomes. We now know, for example, that the health of your gut microbiome is key to your pregnancy health outcomes, and that of your future baby's long-term health.

## DO I HAVE A FERTILE GUT?

**Optimal digestion is evident when you regularly**

- Are able to eat your meals without any abdominal discomfort afterwards.

- Don't experience bloating, wind, gas, reflux, heartburn or gastric pain (and don't take any medication for these).

o   Have one to three bowel movements a day that are well-formed (not loose, runny or hard), are sausage-like (not lots of little balls or small pieces), don't require straining to pass, medium brown in colour and do not contain any blood or mucus.

You are likely to have less than optimal digestion if you don't fit into the above 'optimal digestion' criteria. We often see patients who aren't aware that symptoms such as moving their bowels once or twice a week or regular bloating after meals is a sign that their digestive system is not working optimally and that this may be impacting on their fertility and overall health.

## Susan and Michael's Story

*Susan (29 years old) and Michael (30 years old) consulted the clinic after trying to conceive for two and a half years with three unsuccessful rounds of IVF. Susan had been diagnosed with endometriosis and her IVF specialist had told her that "her eggs were fragmented" (i.e. parts of the cell had broken away and separated from the nucleus).*

*Susan and Michael were highly motivated given their past history and decided to postpone IVF for four months while health issues and nutritional deficiencies were addressed. We identified Susan's digestive discomfort with certain foods as she complained of always feeling fatigued, needing to nap to get through the day and experienced frequent coughs and colds. Blood tests also revealed low vitamin D and iron along with high-fasting glucose levels. In addition, a hair mineral analysis found high levels of copper and slightly raised levels of mercury and aluminium suggesting an increased burden of heavy metals.*

CREATE A FERTILE LIFE

Treatment focused on a gentle detox as well as improving digestive function to improve nutrient levels, reduce inflammation, improve immunity and boost her energy. Susan followed a fertility diet (as outlined in Part 2) in addition to removing foods that were identified as causing her gut disturbance. Supportive herbs and supplements were prescribed to assist general detoxification.

After the detox she reported much better digestion and said her energy had doubled since first coming to the clinic – she no longer needed her naps and was waking after eight hours sleep feeling refreshed and ready to get on with her day. These were great signs her digestion had improved, her blood-sugar was stabilising and her body was becoming more replete in the nutrients she needed. These nutrients would be filtering down to her ovaries and maturing eggs as well.

Michael was found to have low zinc levels and we were concerned about the impact of stress on his sperm health. Thus, specific herbs and nutrients, along with appropriate diet advice were prescribed to help manage stress and enhance sperm and cellular health.

To Susan and Michael's surprise, after three months of working with their naturopath, they conceived naturally. Susan and Michael had a healthy boy, continued with their new healthy lifestyle and came back to see us when they wanted to try for baby number two. They achieved another natural conception and a healthy girl. They have just had their third child, another girl.

Of course, in hindsight this couple wished they'd started off with a healthy pre-conception programme at least four months before even starting trying to conceive. In Susan and Michael's case there were a number of factors dampening their own fertility potential such as understanding about healthy nutrition and how important good digestion is, which resulted in the nutrients needed for building healthy hormones, eggs and sperm.

# WHAT CAN I DO TO IMPROVE MY DIGESTION?

Whilst it is always ideal to consult a health professional to tailor a programme specific for your needs, here are four of the most important things you can do at home to improve your digestion.

## 1. Rest and digest

Relaxation is essential for good digestion, so the first rule of eating is to **make time to eat.**

Eat mindfully, take time to smell the food, savour the flavours and really notice the texture and the different tastes. Eating this way will ensure your digestive juices are flowing. Chewing well and eating slower than usual will allow the feeling of fullness to reach the brain, a signal to stop eating.

When you notice that you feel full, listen to yourself and stop eating. Only eat until full and don't overeat as this puts an extra load on the digestion resulting in digestive discomfort or feeling fatigued after eating. If you find you are an emotional eater, crave the wrong foods or too much sweet or carbohydrate foods then see your practitioner to make a change to habits and thought patterns around food.

## 2. Stimulate your digestive juices

A simple way to assist the body in digesting food is to give some extra stimulation to our digestive juices.

Add a little lemon juice, a teaspoon of apple cider vinegar or your digestive bitters (prescribed by your naturopath) in ½ glass of warm water and sip around 10 minutes prior to eating a main meal. (Note: This may be uncomfortable for those who have high stomach acid; if you notice any discomfort then do not continue).

# 3. Support your digestive elimination

Elimination of waste products is just as important as assimilation of nutrients. If the bowels are moving too fast, resulting in loose stools, then food may be moving through too quickly for your body to absorb all the nutrients. Too slowly, not passing a motion daily can result in a subsequent build-up of wastes in the system as elimination is impaired. This may be adversely impacting your health and your fertility. Aim for one to three well formed, easy to pass bowel motions a day.

> To help to get things moving regularly:
>
> o   Increase water intake (aim for around 1.5 to 3 Litres/day).
>
> o   Include more probiotic and prebiotic foods (e.g. yoghurt with live bacteria, miso, sauerkraut, kefir etc – see below).
>
> o   Increase fibre intake from fruit, veggies, pulses (e.g. chickpeas, kidney beans, lentils etc) and wholegrains (e.g. brown rice, quinoa, rolled oats etc).
>
> o   Avoid foods that are specifically aggravating to you. If you have trouble identifying these, consult with your naturopath and read more about what to do about inflammatory foods in Chapter 15.

# 4. Improve your gut bugs – enhancing your digestive microbiome

Our bodies rely on super bacteria in our digestive system, which have an important role in maintaining and protecting their host organism – us! In fact, about 100 trillion individual bacteria call our intestines home... if we're healthy.

Gut bacteria are integral in moderating our inflammatory processes, and poor gut health may lead to chronic inflammation, which is often implicated in infertility.

## The benefits of good gut bugs

o Help regulate your metabolism; the type of bacteria you carry can go a long way to determining whether or not you are overweight or a healthy weight.

o Assist in the metabolism of progesterone and oestrogen; essential hormones required for conception.

o Supports the production of important nutrients (e.g. vitamin K, B12 and folate).

o Helps support the balance of good bacteria in the vaginal area (vaginal flora) and thus helps reduce the likelihood of bacterial vaginosis (implicated in infertility and miscarriage) and thrush, plus assists in maintaining the correct acid balance (important for sperm survival).

o Plays an important role in our immune health and may impact our allergies or auto-immune health.

o Moderates/reduces inflammation in the body, which is often implicated in fertility.

o Can influence your mental health.

Seriously, there is nothing they can't do... and all these benefits are compromised when our bacteria are not thriving and healthy.

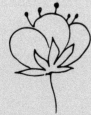

CREATE A FERTILE LIFE

## Why might my microbiome be out of balance?

There are a number of things that contribute to a disharmony of the bacteria in our gut.

o   We inherit our unique gut bacteria population from our mothers, partially influenced by her health during pregnancy, our birth and early exposure to antibiotics.

o   Pharmaceutical medications, including ibuprofen, the contraceptive pill and antibiotics.

o   Prolonged stress.

o   Poor diet: excess sugar, excess alcohol, processed foods, low fibre intake.

o   Gastro and gut infections.

o   Other disrupting factors including pesticides, anti-bacterial cleaners, personal care products and traces of detergent left on our dishes.

## How can I improve my gut bugs?

The upside is that there are many simple things you can do to improve, maintain and look after your friendly bacteria. Bear in mind that you may need a period of restoration to bring you back into balance. The right bacteria are not just 'friendly' but essential for maintaining good health.

o   Invest in a good quality probiotic. Many of the probiotic pills available on the market are insufficient in quality and quantity. Most good probiotics need to be kept refrigerated as they will die when exposed to room temperature for too long. We now have good research to support the use of individual strains for specific circumstances. Consult with a naturopath to ensure you are on the best probiotic for your needs.

o   Choose a good-quality yoghurt that contains live bacteria (not the low-fat, high-sugar variety) with no added sugar. This will be a yoghurt that is plain (not flavoured) and clearly notes the live bacteria it contains, e.g. an organic, no added sugar variety that is 'pot-set' - an environment essential for the bacteria to thrive. Goats, sheep or coconut yoghurt are all good options if you can't tolerate cow's milk.

o   Eat fermented foods regularly, e.g. miso, tempeh, kimchi, sauerkraut, pickles, kefir and kombucha tea.

o   Feed the probiotics with the right foods. As they are actually living organisms, bacteria need food too! Known as 'prebiotics', these are indigestible fibres, commonly found in vegetables including garlic, raw and cooked onion, leek, Jerusalem artichoke, asparagus and green leafy vegetables, plus wholegrains. This will ring alarm bells for those of you with fructose malabsorption or FODMAP issues. If this is the case, consult with your naturopath about how to best provide your bacteria with the foods they need to help them to thrive.

o   Avoid (where possible) those factors known to adversely impact your gut flora (see above 'Why might my microbiome be out of balance?').

o   Avoid foods you know are problematic for you and address underlying factors. If you commonly experience bloating, pain, excessive gas discomfort or poor bowel function, or have been diagnosed with a malabsorption issue or need to follow a FODMAP diet, consult with your naturopath.

# TOP TIPS FOR HIM AND HER

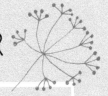

Address any digestive issues such as abdominal discomfort, bloating, excess gas or not experiencing a healthy bowel motion easily and daily.

Relaxation is essential for good digestion, so the first rule of eating is to make time to eat. Sit down, chew well, enjoy the flavours, breathe.

Only eat until full and don't overeat as this puts an extra load on the digestion resulting in digestive discomfort or feeling fatigued after eating.

Activate your digestive juices by enjoying a little lemon juice in warm water or bitters prior to meals.

Improve your gut bugs by including more probiotic and prebiotic foods e.g. yoghurt with live bacteria, miso, sauerkraut, kefir, and vegetables like garlic, leeks and asparagus.

Avoid foods you know are problematic for you, and address underlying factors. If you commonly experience bloating, pain, excessive gas discomfort or poor bowel function, or have been diagnosed with a malabsorption issue or need to follow a FODMAP diet, consult with your naturopath.

If your microbiome is compromised by antibiotics, prolonged stress, high alcohol intake or poor diet then take a quality probiotic supplement.

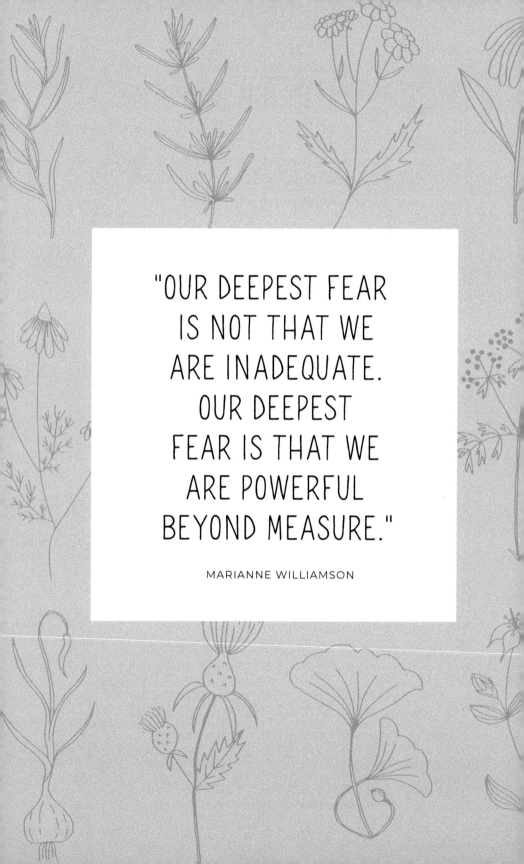

"OUR DEEPEST FEAR
IS NOT THAT WE
ARE INADEQUATE.
OUR DEEPEST
FEAR IS THAT WE
ARE POWERFUL
BEYOND MEASURE."

MARIANNE WILLIAMSON

# PART THREE

# **Flourish**
# Your health, hormones and fertility

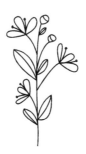

# IN THIS SECTION:

# 13

# Balancing your hormones

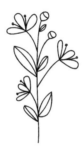

## ARE YOUR HORMONES CONTRIBUTING TO YOUR DIFFICULTY CONCEIVING?

Some women intuitively feel they are suffering some sort of hormonal imbalance. Hormonal symptoms are real, and conditions vary for different women depending on the individual balance between reproductive hormones oestrogen, progesterone, testosterone and prolactin. Other hormones including thyroid, stress hormones such as cortisol and insulin can also play a significant role.

Common symptoms associated with hormonal imbalance include:

- PMS or other cyclic symptoms such as acne, headaches or migraines, tender breasts, mood swings, tiredness, poor sleep, night sweats and food cravings.

- o  Irregular periods.

- o  Short or long menstrual cycles (< 27 days or > 31 days).

- o  Very heavy or very light periods.

- o  Painful periods.

- o  Scant or absent cervical mucus changes with ovulation.

- o  Excess hair growth on the upper lip, chin or jaw-line.

- o  Low sexual desire, vaginal dryness or night sweats.

- o  Conditions including endometriosis, PCOS or other hormonal, thyroid or reproductive conditions.

There are specific types of hormonal imbalances (oestrogen dominance or deficiency, progesterone deficiency, testosterone excess or deficiency, excess prolactin, underactive or overactive thyroid) that you may identify with and we will look at these in this chapter.

Hormones may go out of balance temporarily because of diet or lifestyle issues or it may be caused by a particular condition such as endometriosis. There can be a genetic component, and if you speak to your mother or grandmother you may find they experienced similar menstrual patterns to you.

There are a number of ways that hormonal balance will affect fertility such as influencing when and if you ovulate, it will impact the lining of your uterus and so affect implantation of the embryo; and your hormonal environment will even ensure your follicles mature well to create a healthy egg.

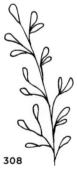

CREATE A FERTILE LIFE

# 10 steps to a more fertile hormonal balance

What we do know is that healthy hormone balance can be achieved and implementing the recommendations of this book will have many women feeling substantially better (whether you have a hormone imbalance or not). Integrating the dietary and lifestyle tips from earlier chapters into your life may be all you need for healthy hormone balance. If you choose to look after yourself well with nourishing food, sunlight, sleep, exercise, consciously avoiding endocrine disruptors (like plastics and fragrances) and managing your stress levels then it will be good for your hormones too!

If you relate to any of these signs and symptoms, support from a naturopath or traditional Chinese medicine (TCM) practitioner at this stage will help facilitate a faster return to a healthy menstrual cycle, optimise your fertility and ensure your body is receiving nutritional support for healthy hormones.

All of these recommendations are extra important if you have recently come off the contraceptive pill or a hormone-based IUD. It may take some time for your body to find its natural hormonal rhythm again.

Here is a quick recap of the basics, which have mostly been covered in detail in Part 1 and 2 but worth a quick refresher, as these are vitally important to restoring hormonal health.

If you have been diagnosed with a hormonal condition, this is all relevant. Keep reading for more specific information for your condition towards the end of this chapter.

# 1. Avoid sugar and refined carbohydrates

To help keep your blood-sugars stable, reducing or avoiding intake of sugar and refined carbohydrates is essential. This is helped by eating plenty of good-quality protein and including good fats in your diet. Blood-sugar balance is particularly important for women with PCOS, and there are some fabulous side effects of balancing blood-sugar including weight management, more energy and lighter, more stable moods. Blood-sugar balance is so important for your reproductive health and fertility that we have devoted a whole section to it! See more in Part Three.

# 2. Fatten up your hormones

Omega 3 fats make healthy cell membranes and allow hormonal messengers to efficiently reach their destination, contributing to healthy hormonal balance. Good fats also help create satiety (a feeling of fullness or satisfaction) and so help to offset cravings for other foods. We also need fats to make cholesterol, which provides the building blocks for all our reproductive hormones. So choose full-fat and avoid low-fat foods and dairy.

Likely your naturopath will prescribe you a quality, well balanced EPA/DHA fish oil supplement too. Quality and correct dose is so important as you will be taking this every day until you finish breastfeeding for best outcomes.

## EAT THESE FATS

Eggs, flaxseeds, pumpkin, sunflower and chia seeds, walnuts, almonds, Brazil and macadamia nuts, full fat yogurt, fish (such as salmon or sardines), avocado, organic butter, extra virgin olive oil and small amounts of coconut oil. Cook with small amounts of coconut oil, butter or ghee and use olive oil only for low temperature frying or cooking.

## AVOID THESE FATS

Processed and baked foods, which are likely to contain trans fats including bought / processed / packaged foods such as muffins, cakes, cookies, pastries, biscuits and chips; milk or poor quality chocolate; fried foods such as hot chips, donuts, deep fried fast foods; processed snack foods such as microwave popcorn and crackers; fatty cuts of meat, especially if not organic, chicken skin; avoid cooking with seed and vegetable oils such as soybean and corn oil; do not use margarine – we prefer organic butter sparingly.

## 3. Poo at least once a day!

A harmonious digestion with good assimilation of nutrients, a balance of healthy bacteria and minimal interruption from bloating, indigestion and other issues contributes much to a healthy balance of hormones. Fibre not only helps to keep you regular, but also binds with excess or expired oestrogen to help the body eliminate it, leading to better overall hormonal balance. If you are not pooing at least once a day, it is likely you are recycling hormones that were meant for excretion, causing unnecessary build-up. So ensure good levels of fibre from vegetables, fruits, wholegrains, nuts, seeds and legumes, as well as pre and probiotics (see below) to keep you regular. If this is not enough, talk with your practitioner about how you can get things moving.

# 4. Make good gut bugs

Getting your intestinal flora right can make a big difference. Have two generous spoons of a natural unsweetened yogurt daily. Consider goats, sheep or coconut if you are sensitive to dairy, or just try adding them for variety and different nutrients. Other good sources of probiotics are found in miso, sauerkraut, kefir, tempeh and kimchi, and can be eaten often.

It is equally important to include prebiotics in our diet. They provide food for our probiotics, and do the wonderful job of stimulating the growth and maintenance of these beneficial digestive flora. Most vegetables act as prebiotics, especially onion and garlic, asparagus, artichoke and greens. Food supplements such as slippery elm, psyllium husks and pectin also act as prebiotics and can be added with lots of water if your digestion is a little on the slow side. You will find much more info on this in Chapter 12.

# 5. Reduce or quit stimulants

Common sense tells us these are an extra burden on our liver, influence our metabolism and stress levels and therefore will have an impact on our hormonal balance. Quit smoking, alcohol, cola/energy drinks and coffee and you will give your hormones a boost.

# 6. De-stress your hormones

Yes, stress again – it literally impacts everything about us. While we know it is unavoidable, we can take steps to manage it better. All reproductive hormones are made from cholesterol and if we are under stress constantly then instead of the cholesterol making progesterone and other reproductive hormones it can be directed instead down the stress-response cortisol pathway. When this occurs, less available progesterone and reproductive hormones can cause irregular ovulation and menstrual cycle and hamper our fertility.

Cortisol also compromises testosterone production in men, leading to low sperm count. We regularly find that our stressed-out male patients have poor semen analysis and low testosterone levels on testing. Often these test results and their fertility improve as we see positive shifts in stress management.

## 7. Improve your sleep

Sleep allows our body to work better on all levels including assisting in hormonal balance. Did you know that sleeping for long enough in a dark enough room is essential for production of melatonin as well as regulating ovulation? Adequate sleep also balances our blood-sugar levels and reduces our stress hormones, which in turn impacts on our reproductive hormones. Have a regular sleep routine and aim for an optimal 7-9 hours a night. Read more on this in Chapter 6.

## 8. Get out in the sunshine

A little-known fact about vitamin D is that, in its activated form, it works as a hormone in the blood. Despite our love of sunny days, it has also been shown to be one of the most common vitamin deficiencies in Australians. Research on vitamin D is growing, and it is being found to have far-reaching implications on many aspects of hormonal health. Your vitamin D levels will influence your oestrogen, progesterone and insulin. Ensure your daily sun-soak with no sunscreen lasts at least 10 minutes in summer and 20 minutes in winter between 11am and 3pm. Make sure as much as possible of your face, arms and legs are exposed. Be careful not to burn; if your skin is pale, you may need to go in the sun in five-minute bursts. In Australia, Vitamin D supplementation is commonly required so do ask your team about this.

# 9. Remove xenoestrogens

Xenoestrogen is a term used for compounds that mimic oestrogen in the body. We have a number of these in our environment that we come into contact with on a daily basis. In fact, you probably have a supply in your bathroom cabinet, your kitchen cupboard or among your cleaning products under the kitchen sink! These are often referred to as endocrine disrupters (the endocrine system refers to the organs that produce and manage all our hormones), meaning that they can adversely impact the health of many of our hormones including our reproductive hormones – for both men and women.

Use glass or stainless steel instead of plastic food containers or plastic drink bottles, choose organic cosmetics, personal care and cleaning products and you are off to a good start in minimising your exposure.

## 10. Get moving and maintain a healthy weight

Did you know that if we are overweight our fat cells can become a secondary source of hormone production? Just another reason why maintaining a healthy body weight is so important – it has a direct influence on hormone balancing. Excess body fat is associated with higher levels of inflammation and higher oestrogen production. The more we have, the more we produce. Conversely, this may be one of the reasons women stop ovulating when they are underweight, as there is not enough of this secondary hormone production for a healthy cycle.

Being overweight or obese also negatively affects male hormones, leading to excess levels of oestrogen and suppressed testosterone. This combination affects not only sperm health, but also contributes to the increased risk of cardiovascular disease in these men.

# Specific hormonal imbalances affecting fertility

We have listed a whole lot of signs and symptoms relevant to different hormonal imbalances throughout the coming pages of this chapter. You are likely going to relate to at least some of them, but it doesn't mean there is necessarily anything drastically wrong. We want to encourage you to take extra care with diet and lifestyle if you spot hormonal issues, as simple changes really can make a big difference. However, we also want to emphasise that many of these imbalances are tricky to determine and extra hormonal blood tests or insight from a professional may be needed. Are the hormones high or low or just low in relation to another hormone? Or are you just more sensitive to hormone changes or levels? It's not easy to categorise as hormones are like a symphony rising and falling and creating their own music which changes throughout the cycle. If, for example, you have high oestrogen, then addressing that can naturally bring progesterone back in balance.

Current thinking suggests that if you suffer from PMS especially mood changes it may be linked to a sensitivity to progesterone and the interaction of our hormones and neurotransmitters like serotonin and gamma amino-butyric acid (GABA). Improvement to symptoms is common with healthy diet and lifestyle changes, as well as specific naturopathic and/or Chinese medicine support. If you suffer from PMS, it is worth trying some good quality, organic chamomile flowers or lemon balm to make a strong pot of tea. They are delicious together or separately too. Drink 3-5 cups daily during your premenstrual phase.

# OESTROGEN DOMINANCE

## Is your body telling you that oestrogen is dominant?

If you have one of the conditions or symptoms listed here, it may be that you are experiencing oestrogen dominance:

o  Abdominal bloating before your period and fluid retention generally.

o  Irregular periods.

o  Pre-menstrual moodiness.

o  Pre-menstrual breast tenderness.

o  Fibrocystic breasts, fibroids, endometriosis or adenomyosis.

o  Pre-menstrual food cravings particularly carbohydrates and sugars.

o  Headaches pre-menstrually or around ovulation.

o  Spotting before your period or within your cycle (always get mid-cycle spotting checked out by your doctor).

o  Large clots during your period.

o  Painful periods.

o  Weight gain around the abdomen and hips or being overweight.

o  Thyroid dysfunction (see below for symptoms of thyroid imbalance).

o  Foggy thinking.

o  Fatigue.

o  Insomnia.

There can be many causative factors for these symptoms but if they seem to fluctuate during the month with your menstrual cycle then it is likely your oestrogen/progesterone ratio is unbalanced with a dominance of oestrogen. The really good news is that by following some of the advice in this chapter you can make some simple dietary and lifestyle modifications that will have great effect on your well-being.

## Rebalance oestrogen naturally

Eating a Mediterranean style diet high in fibre rich foods like fruit, vegetable and legumes is a great start. See Part 2 for more on this. Also, include these two easy ways to help rebalance your oestrogen levels as a focus every day:

A. **Enhance your liver's ability to clear oestrogen from the body.**

B. **Improve your dietary intake of phytoestrogens.**

---

## A. Liver support to enhance oestrogen clearance

In health-food discussions and blogs online, detoxification is an overused term. Here we simply mean optimising our normal digestive system and liver function to enhance their ability to remove wastes and toxins from the body. Our bodies are very clever, and they continue to remove toxins and waste products even when we make poor food choices, drink alcohol or smoke, however, all these things compromise the effectiveness and efficiency of our body's natural functions. Easing the load by reducing or eliminating these things from your daily intake assists in removal of excess hormones (primarily excess oestrogen in this case) and creates more balanced oestrogen and progesterone levels in our body.

If you have started to make changes outlined in this book you may already be noticing the effects of improved waste management and detoxification. Removing coffee, cigarettes, sugar and alcohol from your life takes a huge load off your liver. Removing trans-fats such as margarine, baked goods (biscuits, pastries, chips) and deep-fried foods from your daily diet enhances your liver function even more and will improve your health and fertility on all levels.

Double your benefit by adding nutrients required by the liver for detoxification. Adding a daily veggie juice or green smoothie is a simple way to give your body the nutrients it needs. Cruciferous vegetables contain fabulous plant chemicals called indole-3-carbinol, which enhance DNA repair and are very helpful for the liver in clearing excess oestrogen from our body. This group of vegetables includes cabbage, cauliflower, broccoli, Brussel sprouts, kale and bok choy. Aim to include a cup of these in your diet every day, especially in the week or two before your period. You can add some raw to a green smoothie (although avoid doing so if you have a thyroid problem; see below) but preferably steam for a few minutes or add to stir fries – cooking will also enhance the availability of one of the helpful sulphur-plant chemicals.

Most antioxidants are required for optimal liver function and will also protect your cellular function from any negative effects of detoxification so eat a rainbow of vegetables and coloured fruits. For extra liver and bile stimulation and enhancing gut function and elimination of wastes too, include bitter foods such as rocket, endive or radicchio to salads and squeeze some sour lemon into water to drink before meals. Turmeric is a great spice for liver function so include this along with sulphur-rich foods such as onions, garlic, eggs and legumes.

Finally, the liver requires adequate protein to metabolise oestrogen, so eating protein at each meal is recommended.

## B. Increasing phytoestrogens

Phytoestrogens are plant-based oestrogen-like compounds and when eaten bind to oestrogen receptors in the body. With binding, they produce a weaker oestrogenic affect and thereby act as a hormonal modulator. When oestrogen levels are high, phytoestrogens compete for oestrogen receptors, minimising negative effects (such as PMS and painful periods). When oestrogen levels are low, they can compensate (and benefit conditions such as hot flushes of menopause).

## Foods containing phytoestrogens

One serve of phytoestrogens is equivalent to:

- Half a cup of cooked organic legumes such as lentils or chickpeas (easy to make with a salad of coriander or a mix of fresh herbs, balsamic vinegar, avocado, tomatoes, baby spinach and olives).

- 1 tablespoon of freshly-ground (or soaked overnight) flax seeds (sprinkle on porridge, muesli or add to smoothies).

- 100gm organic tofu (delicious marinated in grated fresh ginger, garlic, soy sauce, brown rice vinegar and sesame oil and baked in the oven).

- 1 cup of soy milk - made from whole, organic soy beans (try making a turmeric latte or include with your smoothie).

- Other foods with good levels include oats, brown rice and wholegrains, sesame seeds, sunflower seeds, green beans, carrots, fennel, peas, cabbage family vegetables and parsley. You can easily include some of these into your diet every day.

## How much should I eat?

If you need it, aim for one serve of phytoestrogens a day throughout your cycle and then increase by up to two serves a day in the week prior to your period. Buy whole organic phytoestrogen foods, especially soybean products such as tofu and tempeh and always avoid soy isolates. If you have any concerns about soy, we have written about this in the chapter Eating For Fertility in Chapter 9 – The Soy Question.

# PROGESTERONE AND POST-OVULATION HORMONAL SUPPORT

The luteal phase of your menstrual cycle begins after ovulation and finishes when your period arrives. This is the time of your cycle that your progesterone rises. After your ovary releases the egg at ovulation, it leaves a structure behind called the 'corpus luteum', which is where progesterone is produced. A healthy egg developed to 14 days before release will leave a healthy corpus luteum and good levels of progesterone will result. Progesterone is the main hormone required to support the development of the endometrium for the best chance of implantation if an embryo is formed. It is essential to support a pregnancy, and adequate levels are especially important in those early weeks after conception. In fact, if you do conceive, the corpus luteum will continue to produce the majority of progesterone until the placenta is large enough to take over production – around 10 weeks into your pregnancy.

The length of the second half of your menstrual cycle from ovulation to your period is ideally around 14 days - the right length of time to create an optimal environment for an embryo to embed and a positive pregnancy result. If your luteal phase is shorter than 12 days, it is called a luteal phase defect, and is likely related to insufficient progesterone production and may potentially indicate a poorer egg quality too.

Charting your cycle is really helpful to determine when you ovulate, the length of your luteal phase and shows signs about the production and stability of your progesterone production too. You can see more information on this in our chapter on Sex and Timing in Part 1 and start charting as soon as tomorrow. No matter where you are in your cycle it will help give information to determine if support is needed for your progesterone levels.

A progesterone blood test will confirm if you have ovulated in that cycle, and also give you an idea if levels are sufficient. The test is called a day 21 progesterone test, but in case your cycle is not a regular 28 day cycle, try to ensure this is done around 7 days after ovulation (e.g. if you ovulate on day 17 then day 24 in your cycle will be the best day for this test, not day 21).

Symptoms of low progesterone can be similar to oestrogen dominance because of the interplay between these two hormones.

## Signs and symptoms of progesterone deficiency

o   Short luteal phase of less than 12 days.

o   PMS - abdominal bloating, mood changes, fluid retention, breast tenderness, headaches

o   Recurrent miscarriage - progesterone helps sustain a pregnancy this is one possible cause.

o   Unexplained infertility.

o   A low basal body temperature during the post ovulation phase and/or a sluggish temperature rise after ovulation (if you are charting your temperature).

o   Irregular menstrual cycle.

o   Conditions like endometriosis, cyclic breast disorders and fibroids (progesterone moderates oestrogen dominant conditions)

There can be other causes for these symptoms and investigation is required to determine the cause before undertaking any specific treatment. Sometimes balancing high oestrogen can result in better progesterone levels after ovulation. Making the diet changes outlined in this book and focusing on the ten steps to a more fertile hormone balance listed at the beginning of this chapter are a good starting point. Check that you're not exercising too much and read through the chapters on sleep or stress if these are likely to be contributing factors. If you suspect that your luteal phase is short or you have low progesterone then visit your doctor for testing and your naturopath for guidance on suitable herbs and supplements to support progesterone production.

# OESTROGEN DEFICIENCY

We have talked about high oestrogen levels, but low oestrogen also needs to be addressed for optimal fertility. If levels are too low then conceiving will be difficult as the endometrial lining of the womb will not develop sufficiently for implantation of the embryo, nor will the follicle grow to optimal size during the first follicular phase of your menstrual cycle. Conditions such as premature ovarian insufficiency, early menopause, low weight and absence of a menstrual cycle all indicate low oestrogen levels. Your doctor can assess oestrogen levels and we also recommend a fertility naturopath or TCM practitioner for further advice.

**Signs and symptoms of oestrogen deficiency**

o Irregular or infrequent menstruation.

o Not ovulating each month.

o Mood swings.

o Low sexual desire.

o Signs of early menopause e.g. hot flushes, insomnia, vaginal dryness, changes in menstrual flow etc.

o Infertility.

o Low oestrogen and high FSH (follicle stimulating hormone) on blood tests on Day 2 of your cycle.

o Thin endometrial lining on ultrasound.

o Low antral follicle count.

o Low Anti-Mullerian Hormone (AMH).

o Bone loss or low bone density.

To help support oestrogen, read back over the *Ten Steps for Hormonal Balance* and add in phyoestrogens which are just as helpful for deficiency as excess. Although fibre is essential, it appears that excessive dietary fibre can in some cases lower oestrogen. If you are underweight then visit a health practitioner to discuss healthy weight gain. Too much exercise can also be a factor here for some.

# Beth's Story

*When Beth first presented she hadn't had a period for over 12 months and was deeply concerned about her health. She worked in a high-stress job as a lawyer and was exercising five to six times a week. She was very slim, pale, and felt like she was in a permanent state of PMS even though she wasn't getting periods.*

*Her diet was hit and miss, with frequent take-away meals after long work days. Beth also had slight yellowing of the whites of her eyes, so we ordered some blood tests to investigate her liver function. Her results came back showing she had Gilbert's Syndrome (a condition affecting the liver), so her script included herbs to support her liver function (an important part of improving her overall hormonal balance).*

*Beth was prescribed herbs to support her nervous system and adrenal glands, and to begin working on improving her hormonal balance. We reduced the intensity of her exercise schedule, and added in good fats, more protein and more wholesome, fresh food to her diet. She began to gain a small amount of weight, such that she now fell within a healthy weight range, and as a result she began to notice changes in her mood, skin, overall energy, and her eyes began to clear.*

*Her periods were yet to return, so high-potency homeopathic medicines were prescribed to try to encourage ovulation. There is very little solid research on homeopathy, but after taking this individually prescribed medicine, Beth began to notice fertile cervical mucus and weeks later had her first menstrual bleed for over a year.*

*Continuing with herbal treatment, Beth's cycle really kicked in and settled into a 30-day pattern. The main factors impacting her hormonal balance had been addressed (poor liver function, low body weight, low oestrogen, nutritional deficiencies and stress), and from there on Beth's cycle remained regular and she was later able to fall pregnant and give birth to a beautiful baby girl.*

---

# TESTOSTERONE EXCESS OR DEFICIENCY

Testosterone is associated with male sexuality, but women also need appropriate levels of this hormone. Testosterone plays a role in our sexual desire, red blood cell production, bone density and muscle mass, and improves our energy levels. So, what do you do if you are suffering from excess or deficient testosterone?

If you experience any of the symptoms listed here, you may want to visit your doctor and ask for your testosterone levels to be checked.

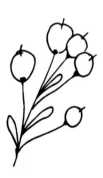

# Signs and symptoms of testosterone excess and deficiency

| EXCESS | DEFICIENCY |
| --- | --- |
| PCOS – if you have been diagnosed with PCOS then you may have excess testosterone. | Low sex drive. |
| Hirsutism – excessive hairiness in women particularly on the chin, upper lip, abdomen (snail trail) and around the nipple (this symptom is the most obvious indicator of excess testosterone). | Persistent fatigue. |
| | Poor muscle mass. |
| | Low mood. |
| Cystic acne. | Fragile bones/low bone density. |
| Increased perspiration. | Poor blood-sugar balance. |
| Irregular periods. | |
| In some cases increased muscle mass and a deepening of the voice. | |

## Balancing your testosterone levels

The most effective way to balance your hormones in the case of excess or deficient testosterone is to balance your blood-sugar. Yes, that old chestnut is the key. When we eat sugars (which includes white, refined carbohydrates) the body releases insulin which helps to move the glucose out of our blood, so it can safely be used for energy. If too much glucose stays in the blood then it can be harmful, and the body responds by pumping out more insulin. This insulin in turn impacts on our ovaries resulting in increased androgens including testosterone. This is another reason why maintaining blood-sugars is so important for hormonal health (see much more on this in the next chapter).

## To reduce testosterone levels

o   Reduce sugars and balance your blood-sugar levels.

o   Eat more phytoestrogens to reduce testosterone by increasing the level of sex-hormone-binding globulin (SHBG). SHBG stops the testosterone from being bio-available in your body. Make sure you eat your daily serve of phytoestrogens such as flaxseeds.

o   If you are overweight then studies have shown that shedding a few kilos may balance your testosterone, which goes for excess and deficient levels.

o   Improve your liver and bowel function to clear excess hormones by adding cruciferous vegetables such as Brussels sprouts, broccoli, cauliflower, cabbage and antioxidant fruit and vegetables to your diet.

## To improve your testosterone levels

o   Eat healthy fats including those in avocados, raw unsalted nuts, olive oil, fish and eggs. Zinc-rich foods are helpful in the production of testosterone. Good zinc levels are found in fish, oysters, beef and lamb, pumpkin and sesame seeds, cashew nuts and spinach.

o    If you do a strength-training program with some weights or resistance bands this will help to build muscle and impact on improving testosterone levels. Find a personal trainer, exercise physiologist or a gym with instructors to put together a routine for you. Eating high-protein foods such as lean meat, eggs, yogurt or nuts and seeds will also help in building muscle.

o   Following our earlier recommendations in Chapters 5 and 6 with good rest, relaxation and sunshine which will also work towards balancing testosterone levels.

Consult with your doctor, and to fast track towards healthier testosterone levels and cycle regularity, consult a naturopath and/ or TCM practitioner to discuss the use of herbs, nutrients and acupuncture to address your symptoms, especially when you are trying to conceive. We find a combined approach helps to re-establish the ovulation/menstruation cycle even faster and generally recommend that women do both naturopathic work and acupuncture concurrently if they can.

# PROLACTIN EXCESS

Prolactin is a hormone produced by your pituitary gland and its main role is to support breast development with a primary function in milk production after child birth. If it is too high during your regular cycle, then it will hamper ovulation and reduce your chances of conception. This is why regular (on demand and at least four hourly) breastfeeding acts as such good contraception after you have your baby, but it is obviously not helpful when you are trying to make one.

## Causes of high prolactin

o   Stress.

o   Medications for example: anti-depressants.

o   Excessive nipple stimulation.

o   Underactive thyroid.

o   Liver or kidney disease.

o   Irritation of the chest wall.

o   Breastfeeding.

o   Prolactinoma (a benign pituitary tumour).

o   Pregnancy.

o   Sometimes no reason can be found. This is called idiopathic hyperprolactinemia.

## Why might your doctor want to test your prolactin?

o  Irregular or absent periods.

o  Producing breast milk even though you aren't breastfeeding.

o  If you have been diagnosed with PCOS.

o  Loss of sex drive.

o  Breast pain.

o  Vaginal dryness.

o  Fertility problems.

o  Unexplained headaches or changes in vision.

If the cause of raised prolactin is benign, treatment may include treating your thyroid (see below), stress management and improving sleep patterns. There are specific herbs that can effectively reduce prolactin levels so seek further help from your doctor, naturopath, and acupuncturist/TCM practitioner.

# 5. HYPER AND HYPOTHYROIDISM

## Is your thyroid over or under active?

The thyroid gland is often overlooked when we talk about reproductive hormones but even if it appears to be within range on your basic thyroid blood test (Thyroid Stimulating Hormone – TSH) it can still be a subclinical cause of hormonal imbalance. Thyroid hormones support metabolism and cell replication, and are therefore key drivers of both egg and sperm maturation, as well as embryonic cell replication. A suboptimal thyroid issue may also affect ovulation and menstrual cycles. It is important to identify if thyroid issues are immune driven (known as Graves' or Hashimoto's disease), as these auto-immune diseases can cause fertility and pregnancy complications of their own, including delayed time to conception and increased risk of miscarriage.

# Sally's Story

*Sally was a 32-year-old woman who presented with a history of unexplained infertility and had recently begun seeing an IVF specialist who referred her to us. Sally had a regular menstrual cycle with some PMS symptoms (anxiety and irritability). She also presented with extreme fatigue (wanted to sleep all day), poor concentration, mild depression and sluggish bowels, which may have been related to recent blood tests showing her thyroid was under functioning. In the last 12 months she had gained 8 kg of weight. Sally's job was not stressful; however, she was feeling the stress of being unable to conceive and feeling tired all the time.*

*Upon assessing her diet, it was clear it was low in protein with no wholegrains and relatively high levels of sugar. Sally started a specific regime, which included herbs, supplements and dietary changes (additional protein, wholegrains, seaweed, fruit and veggies and reduction in sugar) to help support her thyroid function, digestion and nervous system.*

*At Sally's second visit two weeks later, she was feeling better in herself with a little more energy, less anxiety and more consistent bowel motions. After a further four weeks on the regime, Sally was feeling like a different person: her energy had increased (she no longer needed naps during the day), she was feeling happier and had also experienced some weight loss. Additionally, there had been a marked decrease in her PMS symptoms.*

*At Sally's fourth visit (two months later) she announced a natural pregnancy! She needed additional thyroid support to optimise her pregnancy, but her latest blood tests showed an improvement in her thyroid function heading to more normal thyroid levels ideal to support a healthy pregnancy.*

The advice in this chapter on diet and lifestyle are relevant if your thyroid is less than optimal and making some of these changes may be sufficient to balance your thyroid function. If you feel your thyroid may not be optimal then check out the signs and symptoms below. If it relates, ask your GP if it is worth undertaking full thyroid hormone and auto-immune blood tests and get an opinion from a naturopath.

## Symptoms of an overactive thyroid

- Feeling anxious or irritable.
- Tremor or heart palpitations.
- Shortness of breath.
- Increased sweating and intolerance to heat.
- Poor sleep.
- Fatigue.
- Weight loss even though no noticeable dietary or exercise changes.
- Diarrhoea or more frequent bowel motions.
- Hair loss.
- Infrequent periods.
- Problems conceiving or miscarriage.
- May have an enlarged thyroid gland.
- Swollen or red eyes.
- Muscle weakness.
- High basal temperature first thing in the morning.

## Symptoms of an underactive thyroid

o  Low mood or depression

o  Weight gain and difficulty losing weight.

o  Fatigue and excessive sleeping.

o  Feeling the cold, and cold hands and feet.

o  Dry skin.

o  Thinning hair and brittle nails.

o  Poor memory and concentration.

o  Constipation.

o  Fluid retention.

o  Irregular, heavy or prolonged periods.

o  Ovulating late in your menstrual cycle.

o  Low sex drive.

o  Problems conceiving or miscarriage.

o  Hoarse or croaky voice.

o  May have an enlarged thyroid gland.

o  If you have PCOS then it is always worth checking your thyroid function as there is a strong link with hypothyroid or auto-immune thyroid issues and PCOS.

o  Low basal temperature first thing in the morning.

### A home temperature test to assess thyroid function

Your basal temperature – your temperature at rest– can be checked in the first half of your menstrual cycle before ovulation, immediately upon waking. If under-functioning, you will see temperatures regularly under 36.3, and if over-functioning you will see temperatures regularly over 36.9. Re-read the chapter on Sex and Timing in Part 1, which explains charting your menstrual cycle and taking your temperature in more detail. There is a chart in the appendix with a link to a downloadable version for you to use to keep a record too.

## Improving thyroid function

o One of the key thyroid nutrients is iodine, and if your thyroid is over-functioning or you have an auto-immune thyroid condition, you may need to avoid iodine in supplements. If under-functioning increase iodine-rich foods such as fish, some quality sea salt, and add seaweeds (such as wakame, arame, dulse, nori and kombu) to food a few times a week.

o Gluten found in wheat, rye, barley (and lesser amounts in oats) can trigger an autoimmune response and contribute to some autoimmune thyroid problems. Many people respond very well to eliminating gluten in the diet, and we see positive results in balancing thyroid function and increase in energy and well-being in our patients who do this. If you suspect you have a thyroid imbalance try avoiding intake of gluten for a few weeks and notice how you feel. However, make sure you have been tested for coeliac disease prior to starting any gluten elimination. If you have tested positive for thyroid antibodies (especially thyroid peroxidase antibodies) then coeliac positive or not, we suggest that you cut both gluten and casein (the protein part of dairy) for at least 6 months to start to notice an impact on your thyroid antibodies.

o Selenium is a powerful antioxidant and useful in protecting our thyroid gland. Eat more by increasing your intake of Brazil nuts (nuts from Brazil, the USA or South Africa may contain more selenium), snapper and halibut fish, sunflower seeds, organic beef, lamb, chicken and turkey, wholegrains like brown rice, button and shitake mushrooms and garlic.

o Other nutrients needed for a healthy thyroid include tyrosine found in protein foods, iron (get your iron levels checked and supplement if needed), zinc, copper, antioxidants (rich in our fruit and veggies) and omega 3 fats.

- Soy and *raw* cruciferous vegetables like broccoli, kale, cauliflower and cabbage should be avoided if you have an underactive thyroid. If you have an overactive thyroid, making sure you eat one cup a day of these could help.

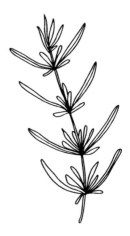

# TOP TIPS FOR HER

As you can see, there are many factors that can contribute to hormonal imbalance but regaining your hormonal health may not be as tricky as it might feel when you are suffering the symptoms. Following our recommendations and getting specific advice for your unique circumstances can produce inspiring results.

Limit or avoid alcohol, coffee, sugar, artificial sweeteners, refined carbohydrates, and stop smoking.

Eat healthy fats daily and remove trans fats such as margarine, baked goods (biscuits, pastries, chips etc) and deep-fried foods from your daily diet.

Go organic.

Have two generous spoons of a natural unsweetened yogurt daily.

Throw out old plastic food containers and store food in stainless steel, ceramic or glass.

Only use BPA-free water bottles, preferably glass or stainless steel.

# TOP TIPS FOR HER

Maintain a healthy body weight and exercise
– a minimum of walking 30 minutes a day and
try to include some weight bearing exercise too.

Seven to nine hours of sleep of a night.

Eat phytoestrogens daily especially if you have high
or low oestrogen. Foods such as organic tofu or tempeh,
legumes, flaxseed meal or LSA mix (avoid tofu and
soy if you have an underactive thyroid).

Get out in the sunshine every day.

For overactive thyroid, eat one cup a day of any or a
combination of these vegetables: cabbage, cauliflower,
broccoli, Brussel sprouts, kale and bok choy. If you have
an underactive thyroid, you should limit consumption
of these foods, especially if raw.

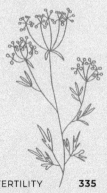

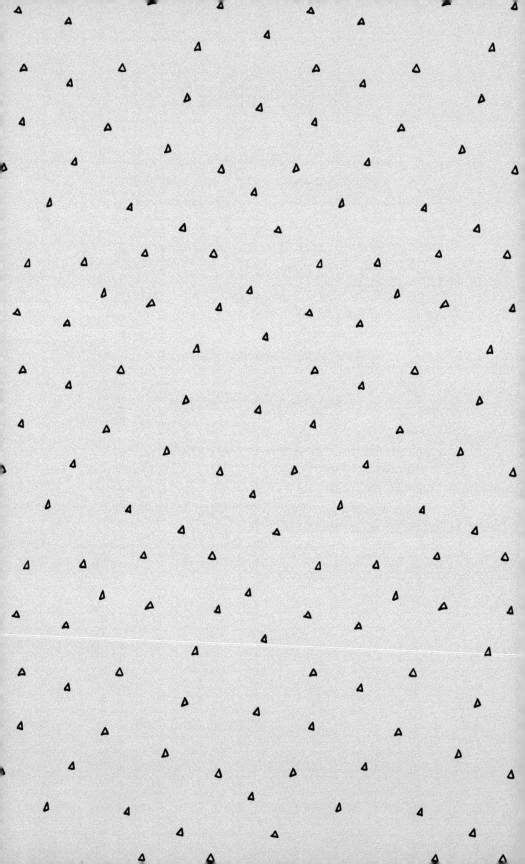

# 14

# Blood-sugar, hormones and fertility

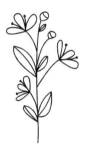

As you've probably already learnt, your diet has everything to do with your fertility. Let's explore more about why your blood-sugar levels matter, especially if you're carrying extra weight, you've been diagnosed with polycystic ovarian syndrome (PCOS), you're a woman with irregular menstrual cycles or a man with poor sperm quality. It is well established that irregular blood-sugar, insulin resistance and diabetes have a negative effect on fertility outcomes for both men and women so it is very important that we address this head on.

## HOW TO IDENTIFY IF YOU HAVE BLOOD-SUGAR ISSUES

Many of us have trouble with blood-sugar levels without really knowing it, and these can cause physiological problems well before your test results will lead your doctor to inform you that you are at risk of developing diabetes. Once you get to this stage, you're well down the path of disease development.

**You are likely to be pre-disposed to blood-sugar problems if you have:**

o   A family history of Type 2 diabetes.

o   PCOS.

o   Experienced gestational diabetes with a previous pregnancy.

**You are likely to be struggling to control your blood-sugar levels if you suffer from any of the following:**

o   Eat a predominantly carbohydrate diet.

o   Have energy slumps in the afternoon.

o   Get regular headaches.

o   Crave sugary foods, cordial or fizzy drinks, chocolate or carbs.

o   Have energy drinks, colas or coffee to give you a lift.

o   Easily become 'hangry' (angry when you're hungry), shaky, or faint.

o   Faint or foggy-brained.

o   An 'apple'-shaped body.

# HOW DO BLOOD-SUGAR ISSUES AFFECT MY FERTILITY?

Blood-sugar issues not only lead to an increased risk of obesity, Type 2 diabetes, cardiovascular disease, dementia and some cancers, your blood-sugar is directly related to many causes for suboptimal reproductive health and infertility as well. There are a number of ways your blood-sugar can create problems with your fertility including impacting your hormonal imbalance and creating inflammation. The good news is that this is totally within your control! What you put in your mouth dictates what happens to your blood-sugar levels on a biochemical level.

As we've already explained, carrying extra weight as either a man or a woman negatively affects your fertility. In fact, one of the main suspected causes of impaired fertility related to weight is the underlying issue of insulin resistance, affecting hormone expression and inflammation. This can lead to compromised ovulation and egg quality in women, and impaired sperm production in men. Not only will managing your blood-glucose levels through diet and exercise help you to lose the extra kilograms but getting your blood-sugar and insulin sensitivity under control will improve your hormones and fertility.

Don't be fooled into thinking that just because you're not overweight that your blood-sugar is spot on. If you tend to crave sweet, sugary or carbohydrate-rich foods, get shaky or irritable if you are late eating or miss a meal then this chapter is still highly relevant for you.

### Do I have blood-sugar issues if I only get sugar cravings before my period?

Many women experience a particular increase in cravings for sugar and chocolate when they are pre-menstrual. Of course, hormones play a role here, and following our advice on balancing your hormones usually helps with these premenstrual sugar cravings. But just as importantly, managing your blood-sugar fluctuations by following the dietary recommendations here will also help to improve your pre-menstrual symptoms, plus benefit your early pregnancy outcomes should you happen to have conceived in that cycle.

## Sugar and stress

Eating excess sugars and refined carbohydrates can also contribute to higher stress levels. Blood-sugar spikes trigger your adrenal glands to produce higher levels of cortisol, the body's primary stress hormone. A common experience when 'quitting sugar' is one of improved stress tolerance and relaxation, plus broader benefits such as concentration and productivity. As outlined throughout this book (and particularly in Chapter 5 on stress) higher levels of cortisol can adversely impact your fertility for both men and women, so breaking the sugar habit is crucial in improving your fertility when you have blood-sugar issues.

## Polycystic Ovarian Syndrome (PCOS)

Some women with weight problems and insulin-resistance issues find they are diagnosed with Polycystic Ovarian Syndrome, or PCOS. This is the most common endocrine disorder affecting female fertility, with 8-13% of women of reproductive age having the syndrome.[169] It seems to have a significant genetic component, and you are likely to find your mother, sisters, aunts or cousins have similar symptoms, or that you have a family history of Type 2 diabetes. But there is no need to despair if you've been diagnosed. Successful management of PCOS is something we regularly achieve in our practice, very often resulting in improvements in symptoms and successful pregnancy within months of treatment.

Common symptoms of PCOS include long or absent menstrual cycles, acne, male-pattern hair growth, weight gain especially around the abdomen and upper body (the apple shape), and a tendency to crave sugar and carbohydrate-heavy foods. PCOS is diagnosed via ultrasound to confirm the presence of multiple cysts on the ovaries, taking a patient history to determine irregular or absent periods and related hormonal signs and symptoms, and blood tests to confirm high testosterone (or symptoms like acne and hirsutism). You only need two out of these three criteria to be diagnosed with PCOS – you don't have to have multiple cysts on the ovaries to have PCOS.[170]

Being a 'syndrome' rather than a 'disease', symptoms and test results vary from woman to woman. It is not uncommon for thin women with irregular cycles to be diagnosed with PCOS, or for women with irregular cycles and multiple cysts to show normal blood-glucose and hormone levels. Clinically, we often find these women present with some of the other secondary symptoms (hair growth, acne), and respond well to breaking their sugar addiction with a low-carbohydrate diet. These women are often told they have polycystic ovaries, but without the syndrome (PCO).

It's important to remember that every woman with multiple cysts and ovulation problems can have a different presentation, and it is unlikely you would have all the signs and symptoms commonly listed.

## The signs and symptoms of PCOS

- Infrequent ovulation and irregular, prolonged or absent menstrual cycles.

- Subfertility and fertility issues.

- Weight gain, especially associated with abdominal fat deposition, but just as often under or normal weight women can present with PCOS. Weight and body-shape changes after stopping the oral contraceptive pill are common.

- Excess dark body hair around the nipple, chest, belly, chin and upper lip.

- Hormonal acne.

- Poor blood-glucose control with frequent cravings for carbohydrates and sugary foods.

- Hormonal imbalance on blood test results may be high testosterone, low sex hormone binding globulin (SHBG), altered ratio of lutenising hormone (LH) to follicle stimulating hormone (FSH), high oestrogen, low progesterone and high blood-glucose and insulin levels.

- Multiple cysts on the ovaries seen on ultrasound.

## What makes a woman susceptible to PCOS?

Unfortunately, you may feel as if your biology is working against you. PCOS is more likely if you have a family history of Type 2 diabetes or if your mother had gestational diabetes when she was pregnant with you. You are also at increased risk of developing gestational diabetes once pregnant and Type 2 diabetes later in life. But it's important to remember that you have some control of your health outcomes at the end of the day. The tools you'll learn to help manage your PCOS symptoms and improve your fertility will also benefit your health long-term and reduce your risk of developing disease later in life.

# OVULATION AND FERTILITY

The major challenge for fertility in these circumstances is related to the irregular cycles. Infrequent, unpredictable or absent ovulation makes timing intercourse for conception very difficult, and egg health may be compromised. This is caused by the underlying hormonal irregularities that we will explain how to improve, but it's also important to remember that if you learn to identify the timing of your ovulation you will be much more likely to conceive more quickly. However, keep in mind it is common for women with PCOS to experience 'bouts' of fertile mucus, which is not always followed by ovulation. Therefore, it is important to make sure you are trying whenever you see fertile mucus throughout your cycle.

# WILL I CONCEIVE?

One of the great misconceptions around PCOS is that you won't be able to conceive at all. You could probably fill a football stadium with the number of 'surprise' babies conceived by women who were told by their doctor they were infertile after receiving a diagnosis. Everyone has heard the stories of the women who hadn't had their period for a year or more, thought they were infertile so didn't use contraception and ended up with an unplanned pregnancy. While these circumstances are admittedly unusual, they do illustrate the fact that once a woman ovulates, she has every chance of conceiving.

Some women with PCOS conceive naturally within a normal timeframe. If you are not one of them then the good news is that with some simple dietary and lifestyle changes you are more than likely to be able to manage your symptoms, improve ovulation, establish a regular menstrual cycle and be able to conceive. Once diagnosed, even medical guidelines prioritise education, self-empowerment, multidisciplinary care, and lifestyle intervention for prevention or management of excess weight.[169] So before heading off to the fertility specialist it is worthwhile taking stock of your health. It will be challenging but making positive changes will be worthwhile and contribute lifelong benefits.

---

## Sarah's Story

*"After getting my first period at 17 years of age and proceeding with a persistently irregular cycle (6 months to a year), I naturally concluded I was not of the breeding kind. This didn't bother me so much at such an immature age, so I wasn't diagnosed with PCOS until I was 23. I was more upset than I ever would have expected.*

*"As you can imagine, I was referred to a gynaecologist who told me to take the contraceptive pill. With no desire to do so, I quickly moved on to see an endocrinologist in Sydney who prescribed a combination of hormones. I took them both for one and a half years (and still feel sick about it) with no period but stopped when I realised one of these medications was given to sex offenders. My periods were very irregular, and I would often skip months.*

"One day in mid-2013 I read an article by a Fertile Ground Health Group naturopath about PCOS, so like all smart people should do, I made an appointment. My first full cycle I had under their care, I had a picture perfect 26 day cycle. They prescribed herbs and some supplements as well as specific dietary changes. The subsequent cycles were anywhere between 32-38 days and I tracked ovulation each month.

"A few weeks prior to my 30th birthday, I decided to try to conceive. I thought it was going to be a long hard road and everyone always says it's better to try sooner rather than later. That month I ovulated somewhere between Day 22-29 and haven't had a period yet! I can confirm from my scan on Tuesday I am now 12 weeks and 5 days pregnant!

"I would like to thank Fertile Ground Health Group for giving my story such a wonderful end."

Sarah went on to have a lovely, healthy baby girl and has since added a baby boy to their family.

---

# WHAT IS ACTUALLY HAPPENING IN MY BODY?

Underlying the symptoms, irregular cycles and hormonal imbalances of PCOS is usually one simple thing: a blood-sugar imbalance. Impaired blood-glucose metabolism in susceptible women leads to the ovaries producing excess androgens, causing a hormonal imbalance affecting fertility. Our aim is to address the cause, so with PCOS we are not just focusing on stimulating ovulation to assist conception. We aim to address the underlying total blood-sugar and hormonal imbalance so that we can not only assist you to conceive by improving your cycles but also improve your skin, weight, and energy. We know this helps you to achieve control over your health, so you are more likely to experience a healthy pregnancy. You can have a reduced likelihood of gestational diabetes, and go on to reduce your risk of diseases associated with PCOS such as obesity, Type 2 diabetes, and cardiovascular disease – for life!

# THE BLOOD-SUGAR/HORMONE BALANCING ACT

If you've worked out you have a blood-sugar issue, here comes the good news. By following our dietary recommendations in Part 2, you'll likely achieve a more regular cycle, an improvement in symptoms and enhanced fertility, along with improving your long-term health outcomes. The following additional recommendations will enhance your success.

## 1. Follow a low glycaemic index (GI) diet

If your weight gain and symptoms are due to blood-sugar levels it is very important that you eat a low glycaemic index (GI) diet to lose the weight. That means plenty of protein, no sugar, no processed carbohydrates, and even limited complex carbohydrates. Your aim is to balance the glucose levels in your blood stream as consistently as possible to prevent them from spiking or dropping throughout the day.

Blood-sugar levels are influenced by what we eat within a matter of minutes.

Sugars and carbohydrates are basically the same thing, just on a different molecular scale. A sugar is a very simple carbohydrate: a carbohydrate is a complex collection of many sugars bound together. The more simple the molecule, the less time it takes to be absorbed from the intestines into the blood stream. The highest GI food is sugar diluted in water (soft drinks and juice fit into this category). Very little digestion is required, so it takes very little time to hit the blood stream. At the other end of the carbohydrate scale, a legume contains plenty of protein and fibre, so it is broken down in the digestive tract more slowly, and the carbohydrates are more gradually absorbed, leading to more balanced blood-glucose levels.

For best results:

o  Combine fat, fibre or protein with a carbohydrate at each meal to help lower the glycaemic index. e.g. eat rice with meat or legumes, or whole grain toast with eggs.

o  Try to eat a good-quality protein at each meal and snack. An emphasis on quality proteins at each meal and snack is integral to balancing blood-sugar. Basically, every time you put something in your mouth it should contain some protein! Be sure to mix it up between vegetable and plant-based proteins so you're not eating meat all the time!

> For more information about GI diets, The University of Sydney has a useful website *www.glycemicindex.com*

## 2. Eat protein-rich meals

For some people eating small, frequent meals also help to manage blood-glucose levels. This can mean eating three smaller main meals and then two to three snacks during the day. And remember each meal needs to contain around a palm size of protein rich foods and all snacks should have some protein too. Research has also shown that women with PCOS benefit from choosing to eat most of their calories earlier in the day rather than later.[171] Have you heard the term 'eat breakfast like a king and dinner like a peasant'?

## 3. Choose your carbs wisely

Choose carbohydrates that contain a lot of fibre, so they are more slowly absorbed.

| CARBOHYDRATES TO INCLUDE | CARBOHYDRATES TO AVOID |
| --- | --- |
| o Vegetables. <br> o Wholegrains e.g. unprocessed brown rice, oats, barley, rye, spelt, wheat, buckwheat, bulgar, millet, corn, quinoa, wholegrain breads (choose quality wholegrain sourdough, sprouted or paleo breads) and pastas (made from the whole-wheat grain). <br> o Legumes e.g. chickpeas, dhal, kidney beans, butter beans, hummus. | o Sugar, including honey, sweeteners, agave, rice syrup. <br> o Commercial/packaged breakfast cereals. <br> o Pastries and cakes. <br> o White processed breads and pastas. <br> o Potatoes. <br> o White rice. |

See more on this in Chapter 9 in 8 Steps to a more fertile diet.

Read labels and avoid all sugar whenever possible. Aim for less than five grams of sugar per 100 grams. Reading labels is an eye-opening experience! It will really help get your sugar down if you try to avoid processed or packaged foods where possible. Individuals with blood-sugar issues and PCOS may benefit from limiting their intake of wholegrain carbohydrates and starchy vegetables to the daytime only and keeping the evening meal to just protein and vegetables.

## 4. Of course, exercise is vital

Regular exercise plays an essential role in blood-sugar control and will help you to manage your weight. A regular exercise routine including cardiovascular and weight-bearing exercise is an integral part of healthy blood-sugar management. The recently updated Australian Government health guidelines recommend physical activity every day, and around two and a half to five hours a week of moderate intensity activity or one and a half to two and a half hours of vigorous intensity physical activity or a combination of both – and so do we. Check Chapter 4 on exercising for a healthy weight to check the guidelines for you which will depend on your Body Mass Index (BMI).

Research has also shown that even just getting up out of your chair each hour and walking around for two minutes lowers blood-sugar levels throughout the day. So be conscious of not remaining sedentary for too long and use every opportunity of incidental exercise to your advantage.

---

### If weight is a problem, it's the first thing that needs to be addressed

First, check your BMI (there are a number of easy BMI calculators online). If you are having irregular cycles, and especially if you've been diagnosed with PCOS, high blood-glucose or insulin levels, and your BMI is above 25, it's time to take action. Research has shown that only 5-10% weight loss can be enough to re-establish regular cycles and enhance fertility outcomes in many women.[172] For example: if you are 80kg then that means a weight loss of four to eight kilograms. We frequently see a return of menstrual cycles in women who lose this amount of weight. With good support this is very achievable.

---

# FASTING – FOOD FAD OR PROVEN BENEFIT?

Have you heard of intermittent fasting? This may also have a significant benefit for individuals with poor blood-sugar control and for many, intermittent fasting contributes to easier weight loss. Two main approaches to fasting have been popularised in recent years.

The '5:2' diet specifically recommends limiting your calorie intake (around 500 for women and 600 for men) on just two of seven days of the week. You can eat anytime of the day so long as you don't exceed your caloric limit – about a quarter of the amount of a regular days intake. This allows you a little more wriggle room on the other days – without going overboard, of course!

The '16:8' diet is practiced every day, with individuals limiting their calorie intake to 8 hours of any given day, ensuring a 16 hour fasting window every 24 hours. For example, you start eating at 12 noon and then stop eating for the day at 8pm. You can vary this to suit your needs e.g. start eating for the day at 11am and stop eating at 7pm. The main idea is to have a 16 hour fasting period regardless of what time you choose to start and stop eating.

These approaches are now backed by research, and clinically we find many patients benefit from adopting a fasting diet. However fasting diets are definitely not for everyone. Consult with your naturopath to consider if this is right for you.

## "I THINK I HAVE BLOOD-SUGAR PROBLEMS, BUT I'M ALREADY THIN"

We hear you. Every day in our clinic we see many individuals who have obvious signs of blood-sugar imbalance or have even been diagnosed with PCOS but are a healthy weight. And even some who have a BMI under 18.5 can actually benefit from putting on a couple of kilograms. For these individuals we recommend following very similar dietary guidelines as blood-glucose levels are just as important, but with a focus on increasing your good fats.

For these smaller women with PCOS, we most often see them achieve their fertility goals when they choose to increase their calorie intake through fats and proteins, but limit sugars and carbohydrates.

These women often have low HDLs (otherwise known as your 'good cholesterol'), which are integral for optimal hormone production and can be elevated by eating good fats. Put simply, this means including foods such as avocado, nuts and seeds, extra virgin olive oil, cold pressed nut oils, fish, and grass-fed meats, as well as a quality fish oil supplement.

If this is you, then it may also be relevant to read our stress chapter in Chapter 5 to help improve your weight too.

## "BUT I CAN'T STOP EATING SUGAR"

While we understand this can be challenging, we find that most of our patients are surprised at how easy it is to break the habit once they are committed to doing so. It doesn't take long before you notice how much better you feel throughout the day, your anxiety dissipates, your energy improves and soon enough you start to desire healthy foods instead of sugar.

## WILL ALL OF THIS REALLY HELP?

We know it will! A 2019 review[173] of high quality evidence concludes that lifestyle interventions (diet, physical activity and/or behavioural interventions) in women with PCOS appear to improve glycaemic results, androgenic symptoms, hirsutism and weight loss outcomes. The role of supplementation in women with PCOS is positive too, showing potential to improve fertility for clinical pregnancy rate. Lifestyle and acupuncture show improvement in glycaemic outcomes and there is some evidence of reduced BMI with lifestyle interventions.

Basically it is what we do when we combine naturopathic support with acupuncture for the best outcomes!

# TOP TIPS TO QUIT THE SUGAR CRAVINGS

o Eat small regular meals. Plan meals and snacks ahead, and always have protein-based, healthy foods on hand.

o Ensure adequate protein intake at each meal, and choose protein-based snacks such as raw, unsalted nuts and seeds, a nut or seed spread (almond butter, tahini) or sardines on bread or toast (wholemeal, mountain, sprouted, nut and seed, paleo, sourdough or pumpernickel bread), natural yoghurt, a slice of cheese, egg-based snacks (e.g. mini quiche, omelette or a boiled egg), miso soup with tofu cubes, hummus or tzatziki dip with vegetable sticks, etc.

o Ensure you are getting enough sleep. Tiredness is one of the key reasons we reach for sugar and willpower is much harder to summon when energy levels are low. Look forward to going to bed early.

o Alcohol and caffeine are not only detrimental to your fertility outcomes, but they also contribute to sugar cravings. Work on eliminating these first.

o Try some exercise when those sugar cravings usually hit. If it is around 10am or 3pm, plan a break and walk around the block, or stand up and do some knee raise marching on the spot or squat jumps to get your blood pumping.

o Try to satisfy sweet cravings with a serve of fruit (two daily) including berries and other low-GI fruits such as grapefruit, cherries, plums and peaches. Add some nuts and seeds, yoghurt or cheese to include protein.

# MORE SUPPORT FOR BETTER SUCCESS

Talk to your naturopath or health practitioner about herbs and nutrients that help to reduce cravings. Willpower is not your only resource and by using herbs and nutrients, we can help to break the cycle of sugar cravings, so you don't have to battle against yourself to fight the urge to eat sugar. Reducing cravings certainly makes it much easier to stick to your new dietary regime and once you are on track, it will feel easy to avoid sugar hits. "No, thank you" you will hear yourself say as your colleagues pass around the lollies or Tim Tams at 3pm.

Many people have found counselling, hypnotherapy or other psychological support very helpful when they are working on weight and food-craving issues. A good psychologist will also be able to help you work out strategies for coping and developing resilience around your cravings. Understanding why you eat what you do when you do can be a real turning point for many people in changing their dietary habits, particularly sticky issues like sugar cravings. Getting help does not mean you have a psychological problem, it just means you are totally committed to making change! Our thoughts and emotions can be our biggest enemy when it comes to food, so please do ensure you are getting adequate support.

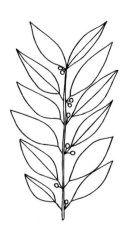

# TOP TIPS FOR HIM AND HER

Calculate your BMI and if you are overweight then ensure you are following a low glycaemic index diet and are exercising regularly enough to lose weight. If you are underweight, still focus on a low GI diet, but also on increasing healthy fats.

Make exercise a part of your normal daily routine, minimum 30 minutes a day.

Avoid sugar, sweet foods, fruit juices, soft drinks, dried fruits, cakes, biscuits and lollies and white carbohydrates.

Avoid alcohol and coffee.

Fill up on foods rich in protein and eat lots of vegetables.

Eat small, frequent meals.

For women, track your basal body temperature to monitor ovulation but be aware that if you have PCOS you may experience regular 'bouts' of fertile mucus before you will see a temperature rise confirming ovulation.

Seek help from a naturopath or health professional if you are struggling to break the cycle of sugar cravings.

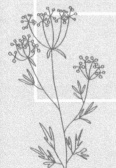

# 15

# Inflammatory conditions and fertility

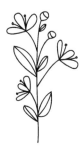

nflammation is emerging as one of the key causes of many types of infertility and indeed much disease in our bodies in the 21st century. Sometimes it is difficult to determine which comes first – does the inflammation trigger the disease or the disease cause the inflammation?

## Inflammatory conditions associated with infertility

o Endometriosis, PCOS, fibroids and pelvic inflammatory disease.

o Recurrent pregnancy loss.

o Egg and some sperm quality issues.

o High natural killer cells.

o Coeliac disease.

o Hashimoto's or Grave's disease.

o Autoimmune conditions.

o Being overweight or obese.

o Inflammatory testicular or prostatic conditions.

o Other inflammatory conditions eg. inflammatory bowel disease.

Inflammation may affect ovarian health and egg development, as well as the vaginal environment, the cervix and cervical fluid, the lining of the uterus and the fallopian tubes. Inflammation impacts negatively on both the health of the sperm and its passage towards the egg along with the chances of the embryo implanting and developing into your healthy baby. If the sperm are affected, they are less likely to make the journey towards the egg, and even if enough do get there, the egg is less likely to favour even one sperm for conception to occur.

So it makes sense to look at the causes of inflammation in both men and women and some simple measures for reducing the amount of inflammation in your body if you are trying to conceive.

## WHAT IS INFLAMMATION?

Inflammation is a natural immune response to irritation, injury, or infection. It is our body's attempt to heal itself as the complex interplay involved in inflammation creates a protective barrier, attempts to expel the causative irritant and brings in all the immune factors, nutrients and hormones in the blood stream required for the healing process. In acute situations like this, inflammation is a wondrous physiological event to be grateful for. Unfortunately for many, inflammation can become prolonged or even chronic, with the same diet and lifestyle factors that plague all aspects of our health and well-being showing up again as a perpetuating problem.

The immune system can also go into overdrive as the process of inflammation causes conditions that lead to more inflammation. In some cases, the immune system can get confused, turn on its own body and start to attack itself in conditions known as autoimmune disease.

# ANOTHER WAY INFLAMMATION AFFECTS YOUR FERTILITY: OXIDATIVE STRESS

Free radicals are tiny molecules in our cells which are a natural by-product of our metabolism. They can be reactive in large numbers and become toxic to cells. Free radicals are both caused by and a cause of inflammation and are linked not just to miscarriage but also other conditions such as endometriosis, obesity, premature ovarian insufficiency, male infertility, unexplained infertility, IVF failure and autoimmune disorders. The damage caused by free radicals is called oxidative stress.

Every part of the reproductive process is vulnerable to this damage: the environment the eggs are developing in, the health, quality and DNA of the eggs, the environment in the fallopian tubes, implantation and pregnancy. Sperm and the DNA contained within are also highly susceptible to free-radical damage during development in the testes as well as on their journey towards the egg within the woman's reproductive system.

Inflammation and oxidative stress are one of the main causes of premature ageing and disease. Affecting every cell in our body, it depletes vitality and energy and is a contributing factor to poor fertility, poor egg and sperm quality and reducing the chances of conceiving a healthy baby.

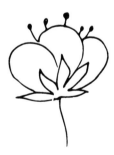

# HOW DO I KNOW I HAVE INFLAMMATION IN MY BODY?

o Generalised fatigue.

o General aches and pains.

o Regular headaches.

o Sore joints including arthritis.

o Sore feet in the morning.

o Sinus congestion/sinusitis/ hay fever/asthma.

o Any pain.

o Digestive problems, e.g. reflux, indigestion, heartburn, bloating, ulcers etc.

o Food allergies/sensitivities or a poor diet.

o Overweight or obese.

o Regularly consuming meals high in calories or saturated fat such as meat, fried foods.

o Over-eating.

o Chronic stress.

o Insulin resistance/Type 2 diabetes/blood-sugar issues.

o Hormonal imbalance if you experience PMS, PCOS, endometriosis, fibroids etc.

o Chronic exposure to environmental chemicals and irritants.

o Drinking alcohol and smoking or other drugs.

o Diagnosed autoimmune disease or autoimmune antibodies.

o Unmanaged hypo and hyper-thyroid.

As it can affect every cell in your body, chronic inflammation and the associated oxidative stress increases your risk of developing other health conditions later in life, like heart disease, Type 2 diabetes, cancer, and is a big contributing factor in weight gain and obesity.

# THE FERTILITY LINK BETWEEN INFLAMMATION, IMMUNITY AND AUTOIMMUNITY

While the research is hotly debated among fertility specialists, autoimmune diseases have become increasingly linked to reduced fertility and infertility and are usually investigated when a couple have experienced recurrent miscarriage (more than three), been put in the 'unexplained infertility' category, or where there is a history (including family history) of autoimmune disease. There are over 100 autoimmune diseases including: Type 1 diabetes, Graves and Hashimoto's disease (both affecting the thyroid), anti-phospholipid antibody syndrome, coeliac disease, inflammatory bowel disease (including ulcerative colitis and Crohn's disease), multiple sclerosis, psoriasis, scleroderma and systemic lupus erythematosus.

When autoimmune disease is present, the body's immune system may be directed against hormones, clotting factors or reproductive tissue itself, such as the ovaries or testes. Inflammation and cellular damage are a part of autoimmunity that can impact on reproduction and reduce a couple's chance of conception. An overactive immune system is thought to be a possible reason for some recurrent miscarriages. For example, Antiphospholipid syndrome (APS) is one of the more common causes of recurrent miscarriages. APS is a condition where normal blood clotting is affected by the body's own immune system creating antibodies to clotting substances. Having this condition may reduce the chance of embryo implantation and pregnancy or if a conception happens a blood clot may form in the placenta and increase the risk of miscarriage.[4]

In other cases of autoimmunity where anti-nuclear antibodies (ANA) or uterine natural killer (NK) cells are high or where other autoimmune factors are at play, an over active immune system may be directed against the endometrium or even reject the developing embryo as if it were a 'foreign' substance or an infection.[174] In these instances the usual chain of events in pregnancy where part of the immune system is dampened down to protect the foetus may not happen and sadly a pregnancy loss may occur.

# The 5-step process
## to reduce inflammation and improve your fertility

## 1. GET TESTED AND GATHER YOUR TEAM

It is important that you discuss with GP, gynaecologist or fertility specialist tests for immunological/inflammatory issues if they are of concern due to family history, or you experience any or a few of the indications listed previously.

If there are any indications that you have an autoimmune issue, it is vital that you consult with an experienced fertility naturopath or Chinese medicine practitioner who can work alongside your medical team for the best outcomes for your fertility. Diet and lifestyle measures impact hugely on this picture, and can turn things around if addressed with rigor. There are also many additional effective herbal and nutritional treatment considerations if you do test positive for any autoimmune factors.

It is highly supportive and effective if your health team are working together and have an understanding of all of the prescription and over the counter medicine or supplements you are taking (no matter how seemingly benign) as there is potential for interaction that needs to be considered. For instance, do you know you can't consume green smoothies, grapefruit or cranberry juice every day if you are on warfarin without needing to reduce your dose? Or that green smoothies containing raw kale may be a problem if you have Hashimoto's or hypothyroidism? Research and health-care team support is very important with these kinds of conditions.

## 2. GET ON TOP OF YOUR STRESS

The immune system responds with inflammation to psychological irritation and trauma as much as physical injury. Cortisol, the major hormone associated with stress is a leading cause of inflammation and when chronically raised it can cause significant dysfunction in the body. There are many things you can do, but the first and foremost thing to accurately assess is the impact of stress on your body. We have discussed this at length in our chapter on stress (Chapter 5). Simply getting your quota of eight hours sleep a night and getting out in the sunshine daily for 10-20 minutes will help to reduce stress, reset your immune function and reduce inflammation.

## 3. MOVE YOUR BUTT

Regular exercise helps our bodies to process stress by using up the stress response appropriately. Your body does not know the difference between different sources of stress. Whether it is a sabre-toothed tiger or a major work crisis, it is all the same from a hormone point of view – so get your boxing gloves on! Skip, run, fast walk, dance, swim, ride... whatever you please. Getting your body moving, your heart pumping and your sweat flowing definitely helps metabolise cortisol out of your system and will even provide you with some uplifting feel-good hormones like endorphins! Exercise also stimulates our immune system, in turn helping the body to 'mop up' any excess inflammation.

# 4. EAT MORE ANTI-INFLAMMATORY FOODS

Follow our recommended diet as outlined in the food chapters (Part 2) with particular attention to increasing your consumption of anti-inflammatory foods and foods high in antioxidants to combat oxidative stress.

## Foods that may decrease inflammation and oxidative stress when consumed daily

- Colourful organic vegetables and fruits, green leafy vegetables, pineapple (including the bromelain-rich core) and papaya.

- Healthy fats particularly foods rich in omega 3 – oily deep sea fish such as salmon, sardines and herring, plus almonds, chia and flaxseed, walnuts, pumpkin seeds.

- Herbs and spices such as turmeric, cinnamon, ginger, basil, coriander, mint and parsley.

- Onions and garlic (use both cooked and raw).

- Herbal teas such as chamomile, licorice, lemon balm, nettle, rooibos and ginger.

While including the above food groups in your daily diet, avoid the following foods, ingredients and chemicals that increase inflammation and oxidative stress.

## Foods that may increase inflammation and oxidative stress

- Those known to commonly cause reactive inflammation in many people. See the suspect line up of foods over the page under The Fast and Challenge Diet.

- Processed, packaged and pre-prepared foods – and especially fast food outlets thanks to the harmful oils, sugar and artificial sweeteners, food additives, and a whole host of nasty ingredients contained in their ingredient lists.

- Fried foods get a special mention. Hot and cold chips, fries, crisps, onion rings, hamburgers. They speak for themselves really!

- Cut down on foods and oils containing omega 6 fats – safflower, sunflower, soy, corn, and sesame.

- Cut out sugar in all its forms. Also watch out for high fructose corn syrup, a highly-refined product used in soft drinks and many processed foods. Sugar can creep in to even the healthiest diet – think honey in tea/chai, dried fruit with nuts, fresh dates, maple syrup, even fruit yoghurt! It all adds up to aggravate inflammation.

- Synthetic sweeteners made from saccharin or aspartame are linked to many serious health conditions. These are the products often labelled as 'diet', 'low joule' or 'no sugar'. Don't use them.

- Cut out caffeine in coffee, chocolate and any energy drinks. Apart from the sugar usually contained, caffeine has been shown in research to directly exacerbate the damage caused by inflammation.[175] As it also drives up our adrenals and cortisol levels (stress response), it has a double-whammy effect and should be avoided.

- Cut out alcohol in all forms because you are trying to conceive, and it's also a major contributor to inflammation.

- Artificial colours, flavours, preservatives. Read your labels carefully if you are choosing to eat food in a packet.

- Meat is on the list, too. While you don't necessarily have to go vegan or even vegetarian, plant-based diets are much higher in anti-inflammatory compounds. In general, don't make meat the main part of your meal. Trim the fat off any meat, especially red meat or non-organic meat. Consider meat an addition of flavour and protein rather than the centre of the meal and aim for several meat-free meals every week.

## Getting rid of inflammatory foods from your diet

Your diet plays a powerful role in promoting or preventing inflammation, oxidative stress and supporting your immune function. Especially when combined with cutting your stress levels and moving your body, changes to your diet can make a big difference to your levels of inflammation.

Research suggests that many common inflammatory conditions may be affected by certain food allergies, intolerance or sensitivity reactions that contribute to inflammatory symptoms. Aside from inflammation and pain directly affecting the gut, you won't be maximising nutrient absorption from food or supplements, contributing to widespread deficiencies.

Eliminating the suspect foods from your diet can significantly reduce common inflammatory symptoms and improve your general health and well-being.

And it is easier than it sounds! The good thing is that with a bit of detective work, we can identify the sensitivity signs to particular foods or food groups.

If you are finding it difficult to identify what is triggering your symptoms, think about the food group you love the most. What would you rather tuck into above all else? A platter of cheese or an ice-cream? You may be looking at a dairy sensitivity. Vegemite on toast, beer or blue cheese? You may be starting to suspect yeast. Pasta, bread, cakes or pastries? We are thinking wheat or even gluten might be a problem for you. Interesting isn't it that what you can't live without may be the thing that is reducing the quality of your life!

The addiction to foods you are sensitive or allergic to stems from the fact that the cascade of reactions the particular food group sets off for you includes histamines – a hormone that your body can start to crave like any addictive substance. This sets up a craving/satisfying/ symptom-aggravating cycle that can be hard to identify and break. Getting experienced support is helpful in identifying your food sensitivities and developing strategies and alternatives so you can stay away from them.

## 5. IDENTIFYING THE SUSPECTS – THE FAST AND CHALLENGE DIET

In a fast and challenge diet, we support you to eliminate one suspected food group at a time. For instance, if it is cheese and ice-cream you crave (or suspect), we would ask you to eliminate all dairy products for three weeks. This includes milk (and café lattes!) cheese, butter, yoghurt, ice-cream, cream and dairy-based chocolates. Many cakes and biscuits will have to go as well. For the first few days, this will be really hard, as your body fights the cravings for the histamines and pulls on your willpower to give in and have a glass of milk. You may even experience some detox reactions like headaches or fatigue. After the first week though, most people find that – if they have chosen the right food group to eliminate – the cravings stop and they start to feel some improvements in their signs or symptoms.

At the end of the three weeks, it is time for the challenge. We want you to have a full day's enjoyment of your suspected food group. To continue with the dairy example: milk on your cereal, cheese in your lunch and a yoghurt after dinner. If you have honestly eliminated dairy over three weeks, you should know within 24-48 hours (but often immediately) of reintroducing the food what the reactions are for you. You may notice an improvement in your symptoms or your energy or general health within the fast/elimination time and then an aggravation of the inflammatory symptoms when you reintroduce the food group: fatigue, headache, digestive discomfort, diarrhoea, constipation, sinusitis, joint pain or other reactions you didn't expect.

Or you might come down with a cold as your body struggles to cope with the load. If you don't react, it's time to try another food group. But watch carefully. Many people find they don't want to reintroduce the food they eliminated as they feel so much better without it.

## Step 1: Eliminate the suspect foods

Eliminate the suspect food/food group completely for three weeks. It is easier to try one food group at a time, but you may be curious or feel committed to try more and get it over with.

## Step 2: Challenge

At the end of the three weeks, it is time for the challenge. Reintroduce the suspect food for one day in decent quantities. Only one food group at a time if you have fasted from more than one. Watch for signs and symptoms over the following day.

## Interpreting your fast and challenge results

**LIKELY RESPONSE INDICATING AN INFLAMMATORY REACTION**

Initial response (usually occurs within the first 24 to 36 hours):

- Aggravation of the inflammatory symptoms.
- Fatigue.
- Headache.
- Digestive discomfort or pain.
- Sinusitis or joint pain.
- Other reactions such as nasal congestion (or a cold), runny nose, sneezing, skin rashes or breakouts, change in bowel movements.

**LIKELY RESPONSE INDICATING NO REACTION**

- You don't feel any different!
- If this is the case, then repeat the fast and challenge with a different suspect.

### Identifying the suspect foods

Working out what foods may be an issue for you can be difficult; however, there are certain foods more likely than others to be associated with an inflammatory reaction.

## Suspect food groups – a good old-fashioned line up:

- Dairy – milk, butter, cheese, yoghurt, ice cream, frozen desserts, cream, sour cream, milk chocolate, whey, milk powder, and many cakes, biscuits and processed foods.

- Soy – soy milk, tofu, tempeh, edamame, miso, soy sauce (tamari, shoyu, teriyaki), imitation meat products, TVP, isolated soy protein, many processed foods (you must read labels).

- Wheat – bread, pasta, bulgar, couscous, khorasan, kamut, burghul, farro, freekeh, spelt, semolina, triticale, flour, scones, muffins, pancakes, cookies, cakes, wheat germ oil, wheat grass, glucose syrup, soy sauce, processed meats and sauces like gravy.

- Gluten – wheat (including all above), rye, oats, barley, and all food derived from these sources. Read labels carefully!

- Eggs.

- Corn.

- Nuts, especially peanuts.

- Shellfish.

- Solanaceae / nightshade family: potatoes, tomatoes, capsicums/peppers, eggplants, chillies, goji berries, tobacco.

# THE ANTI-AGEING BONUS

The benefits of an anti-inflammatory diet and lifestyle regime extend beyond creating healthier eggs, sperm, and embryos. Alongside creating an optimal developmental environment, this approach comes with the added bonus of being anti-aging too!

Inflammation and free-radical damage or oxidative stress causes cells to function poorly and die prematurely. Not only will your reproduction reap the benefits, your whole body will improve in function as your immune system is freed up for regular work, your cells are repaired, your organs function more healthily, your skin and eyes are brighter, and you feel more vital in general. You will also find very similar recommendations for cancer prevention and treatment of most chronic health problems.

So, start now! Your body will thank you in many more ways and have you well on the way towards conceiving your healthy baby. And if an anti-ageing bonus piques your interest, read on for more in our next chapter on Beating Biology!

# TOP TIPS FOR HIM AND HER

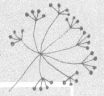

Make a list of all your symptoms and ask your health team for their opinion to determine if inflammation is playing a role in your fertility problems.

Get serious about managing your stress!

Aim for seven to nine hours of sleep every night.

Get out in the sunshine every day.

Move your butt!

Eat more colourful organic vegetables and fruits, oily deep-sea fish (such as salmon, sardines and herring), almonds, flaxseed, walnuts, pumpkin seeds, herbs and spices (such as turmeric and ginger, basil, coriander, mint and parsley), onions, garlic and herbal teas (such as chamomile, licorice, lemon balm, nettle, rooibos and ginger).

Avoid sugar, alcohol, caffeine, fried or processed foods and artificial colours, flavours and sweeteners.

Aim for several meat-free meals each week and when eating meat look for organic or grass-fed meats.

Fast and challenge: identify suspect inflammatory foods in your diet and then remove them for three weeks. Introduce them one by one and monitor your response to identify foods that may be causing inflammation in your system.

# 16

# Beating biology

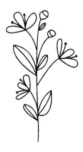

## HOW DOES AGEING AFFECT EGG AND SPERM QUALITY? CAN ANYTHING BE DONE ABOUT IT?

Age is the single biggest factor affecting a couple's chance of conceiving, which can be frustrating because it feels like the one thing we can't do anything about, right? Well, not exactly. While some of the facts are hard to hear, there can be an upside. Knowledge is power so if age is likely to be a consideration for you, read the hard facts below and continue reading to see what you can do to help your fertility despite your age.

While the tabloids love to tell us about famous women having babies well into their 40s, what they fail to tell us is that in many cases a (younger) donor egg has been used and sometimes even a surrogate mother. The fact is that a couple trying to conceive by this age are much less likely to experience a healthy pregnancy and birth. Age does indeed have an impact on fertility for both men and women. The good news is that egg health can be influenced positively by improving ovarian health and the follicular environment your eggs are developing in. Sperm health, too, will benefit from healthy diet and lifestyle changes.

Women are essentially born with all their eggs. In fact, the number peaks at about 18-22 weeks in utero – before she is even born – with numbers reaching six to seven million, which decline to around one to two million oocytes by birth. There is a further decline by the completion of puberty to a total of around 250,000 eggs in both ovaries – and at this stage most of us are not even considering conceiving for many years to come.

For a long time, there has been a commonly-held belief that the health of your eggs is determined well before you are born. This concept is slowly getting turned on its head as we now know that egg quality can be influenced in the 100 days before ovulation whilst they are maturing. However, it does remain true that age is a big factor in your chances of conceiving a healthy baby, with statistics showing a decline in a woman's fertility from 35 years old, and a steep drop in chances after 41.

While there are examples of men fathering children into their golden years, it is a mistake to believe there is no impact of ageing on a man's fertility. Most importantly, a man's age impacts on the quality of sperm, reducing a couples' chance of having a healthy child and increasing their risk of miscarriage.

When it comes to age – for both men and women – it is not just biology but also the accumulation of your lifetime that catches up on the health of the eggs and sperm. Poor eating habits and lifestyle choices, cigarette and passive smoking, alcohol or other drugs, nutrient deficiencies, hormonal imbalances, reproductive illness, being overweight, obese or underweight, acute health conditions, acute and chronic stress, exposure to harmful environmental substances... the list goes on and of course continues to build as we age – unless we do something about it!

Focusing on egg and sperm quality (health) is essentially what preconception care is all about. It is important for all couples trying to conceive to do it consciously, and it is especially important as we age. The main message here is that you need to start now, with even more focus and attention on all the recommendations for preconception health. For couples who have sadly experienced miscarriage or conceived babies with chromosomal issues in the past, working on egg and sperm quality is essential to improve the chances of healthier outcomes for the next pregnancy.

# JUST IN CASE YOU DON'T ALREADY KNOW THESE STATS

The average age of menopause (defined by the absence of menstrual periods for 12 months) is 51, and usually occurs somewhere between the mid-forties and early sixties for the majority of women.[176] At an individual level, fertility dramatically declines around 10 years before the final cycle though, so some women find themselves struggling to conceive before they even consider age to be a factor. Hindsight is a wonderful thing. Whilst the age your mother went through menopause may provide some indication as to what age you may experience menopause, it is not a definite predictor in determining when it will occur for any individual women.

Fertility peaks between the late teens and early 20s. Statistics show a woman's fertility starts to decline in her early 30s, speeding up after 35. At 30 years old she has a 20% chance of conceiving on any cycle. By the time she is 40, her chance of conception each month is down to five per cent – whether trying to conceive naturally or through IVF.[177]

## The impact of age on fertility [178]

| FEMALE AGE | CHANCE OF CONCEPTION WITHIN 12 MONTHS |
|---|---|
| 25yo | 90% |
| 35yo | 75% |
| 40yo | 50% |
| 45yo | 10% |

## More age-related facts for women[177]

o  As age increases, the risks of other disorders that may adversely affect fertility, such as fibroids, tubal disease, and endometriosis, also increases.

o  Women with a history of prior ovarian surgery, chemotherapy, radiation therapy, severe endometriosis, smoking, pelvic infection, or a strong family history of early menopause may be at an increased risk of having a premature decrease in the size of their follicular pool and decline in fertility.

## If she does conceive[179]

o  More than half of women aged over 42 experience pregnancy loss and the risk of miscarriage is higher than the chance of live birth over 40 years of age.

o  Over 35 years of age, the risk of stillbirth is two and a half times higher, and over 40, the risk is five times higher than for women under 35 years old.

o  The risk of chromosomal abnormalities in the baby increase from 1 in 385 for women under 30 to 1 in 63 for women over 40.

o  Older women are considered to be at increased risk of pregnancy complications and higher risk during birth including gestational diabetes, placenta previa and placental abruption.

# THE IMPACT OF MEN'S AGE ON FERTILITY

Men should also know how ageing affects their sperm and the potential health implications for their child if they father a child later in life.

o   There is a continual reduction in the volume of semen and sperm motility and structure between 20-80 years of age.[180]

o   It takes longer to get your partner pregnant – in fact if you are over 40, it is 30% less likely that you will conceive compared to men under 30.[181]

o   It takes five times longer to conceive with a man who is over 45 compared to a man under 25.[181]

o   Sperm DNA fragmentation and mitochondrial damage worsens with age.[161]

o   Pregnancies conceived with men aged over 40 are 60% more likely to miscarry than from men under 30.[182]

o   Men over the age of 50 have almost twice the risk of miscarriage and stillbirth.[182]

o   Whatever the age of the mother, miscarriage is more likely if the father is over the age of 45[180]

o   Children born to fathers over the age of 40 have five times the risk of developing autism spectrum disorder compared to fathers under 30, and more likely to suffer mental health issues and learning difficulties.[180]

o   The risk of schizophrenia doubles when fathers are between 45-49 years of age, and triples if over 50.[183]

# THE IMPACT OF AGE ON IVF

While IVF is increasingly thought to be the saviour for fertility problems including age, the chances of conceiving with IVF are also significantly reduced:

o    The latest data for IVF success in Australia and New Zealand for all fresh cycles shows a 28% live birth rate for women under 30, 25.5% for women aged 30-34, dropping to 16.7% for women 35-39 and 5.6% for women aged 40-45.  Women over 45 only have a 0.6% chance of taking home a baby.[184]

o    The risk of not having a baby is more than five times higher if the male partner is over 41 years old.

o    ICSI, an IVF technique thought to overcome the issue of sperm defects, which are more common in older men, carries a higher risk of fertility problems in the offspring conceived with this technique (inserting the sperm into the egg).[185]

## IS IT POSSIBLE TO REWIND THE TICKING CLOCK?

---

## Naomi's Story

........................................................................................

*Naomi first came to the clinic when she was 42 years old – a single woman commencing IVF treatments on her own, using donor sperm. She had already undergone two stimulated cycles without success. Naomi was achieving reasonable egg numbers for her age (six to eight eggs), but her embryo quality was poor, and she had had no successful transfer.*

*We worked with Naomi for the next two years as she went through regular cycles, and even though a lot of work and time went* to improving her health, she was feeling worse and worse with each cycle, suffering from chronic constipation and worsening anxiety. Naomi was consistently told by her doctors that the issue was her age (which is a very reasonable assumption), and that her best option was to continue with back-to-back treatments as regularly as she could to improve her chances.

By the time Naomi turned 44, she'd had enough. She'd put on 10kg, felt bloated, anxious and completely exhausted. She decided to take six months off IVF before doing one last cycle, as she knew her chances were now very slim. In this time, focus shifted to weight loss, exercise, reducing anxiety, digestive health, whilst the entire time working towards a healthy hormonal cycle and improved egg quality with herbal medicine and nutritional supplementation.

At 44 and a half, Naomi had lost the 10kg, was 'glowing', felt much better in herself, and all her physical symptoms had improved markedly. She commenced her final stimulated cycle, and for the first time achieved a Day 5 embryo transfer. Naomi waited nervously for the two-week wait results, anticipating spotting and cramping, as she had experienced many times before. But the symptoms did not appear, and at her two-week wait blood results, she achieved her first positive result.

Naomi went on to have a relatively healthy pregnancy, and now has a gorgeous two-year-old son to show for all her hard work.

---

## REDUCING YOUR 'BIOLOGICAL AGE'

While there are no magic potions to halt the advance of age chronologically, with most forms of wellness medicine we actually do have the opportunity to reverse our biological age at a cellular level (where it counts!). By making healthy choices, removing harmful wastes and 'toxins' with gentle detoxification and cleaning up our lifestyle (quit smoking, alcohol and any other drugs), improving circulation to the ovaries and testicles (with regular exercise, good hydration, acupuncture), improving nutrition to the developing eggs and sperm (by eating well and taking appropriately-prescribed supplements), and optimising hormonal health.

The health of our eggs and sperm (and indeed all of our cells in our whole body) can actually improve rather than deteriorate. We see the changes most obviously with couples doing IVF as the quality of the eggs and numbers of healthy sperm, the number of eggs fertilised by sperm and the number of viable healthy embryos can and do improve after doing this work.

Women are commonly told by their doctors or fertility specialist that their eggs are too old if they are having trouble getting pregnant past the age of 35. It is not true to say that the health of the eggs is the only factor, as the health of the sperm contributes significantly. It is also not true to say that either cannot be influenced in any way, but it does take time and commitment.

Science is catching up with these recommendations too. For a long time, it was believed there was very little chance to influence fertility positively, especially for women and egg health. But new research is consistently emerging to support what we have always said about the benefits of improving your health as much as possible across all parameters.

Next, we'll delve into the fascinating science about your cellular DNA, telomeres, mitochondria and reactive oxidative species if you are not convinced yet!

# WHY DOES IT TAKE SO LONG?

While we are born with the basic cells that will eventually form our eggs, these primordial follicles do not in fact contain eggs ready for fertilisation to make your baby. They must go through a stage of maturation over many months, with a period of about 100 days where you have the opportunity to influence the health and development of your ovaries, follicles, and the eggs maturing and growing inside. Sperm also undergo a process of development ready for ejaculation over nearly 90 days during which they are very sensitive to the environment they are developing in. If a man has been exposed in the past three months to acute things like an infection or fever, or has recently been training intensely for say a marathon, we can really see a significant drop in the numbers of viable sperm compared to a three month period of healthy living. Does this help to make more sense of why we recommend you work on your health for at least three months prior to trying to conceive?

# WHY DOES EGG AND SPERM QUALITY DETERIORATE WITH AGE?

As we have previously mentioned, it is the accumulation of damaging lifestyle factors that age us and our eggs/sperm. All the factors listed below affect our immunity, nervous system, hormonal balance, dry out our membranes, create increased, unnecessary physiological stress and other effects that cause us to age more rapidly. All our cells are affected right down to our DNA. For example, it is possible that a woman can appear peri-menopausal (hot flushes, irregular periods, dry skin, hair and nails, night sweats, etc.) but is really just affected by lifestyle factors and hormonal imbalances that can be repaired with time, attention and commitment. Addressing the issues that are directly responsible for your ageing are of primary and vital importance to the vitality of your whole organism, particularly the cells of reproduction – your eggs and sperm.

# Timeframe for egg and sperm maturation/production

Eggs take around 100 days to mature (i.e. the egg released this month during ovulation will have started maturing three to four months ago).

Sperm take nearly 90 days to be produced from scratch to the time they are ejaculated (i.e. the sperm trying to fertilise an egg this month will have started to be produced three months ago).[186]

During this three to four-month window, you can influence your egg and sperm health positively or negatively. While many couples affected by the age factor are not in the position to wait another three months before trying, individual factors will vary, and it is worth consulting with a natural fertility expert as soon as possible to assess your need.

Where necessary you can certainly continue conception attempts while following our recommendations. While we don't recommend heavy detoxification programs for women whilst trying to conceive, every menstrual cycle is an opportunity to work on the health of your eggs to come. Once you start trying to conceive, if you are unsuccessful on any one cycle, is it helpful to know that your body is already working on its backup plan. The hormones acting on this cycle are also acting on eggs waiting in line behind, preparing, nourishing, maturing, and getting ready for ovulating healthier eggs in following cycles.

Similarly, for men, the development of sperm can be impacted at all stages of development over this time. None of your good efforts at this stage are wasted. Your bodies are preparing for numerous possibilities. Clever aren't we!

# LIFESTYLE FACTORS ADVERSELY AFFECTING EGG AND SPERM QUALITY

o Smoking increases the age of your ovaries dramatically. Research has shown that smoking reduces fertility and reduces a woman's ovarian reserve.[78,187] Needless to say, it is a disaster for developing sperm also.

o Alcohol.

o Caffeine.

o Low-fat diet.

o Unhealthy fats.

o Processed foods.

o Excess sugar.

o Exposure to pesticides, GMO, antibiotics and hormones in non-organic food.

o Exposure to hormone disruptors such as BPA in plastics and phthalates in cosmetics, cleaning products etc.

o Exposure to radiation sources such as mobile phones, laptop computers, Wi-Fi, bluetooth etc.

# WHY AGEING SEEMS TO BE SUCH A PROBLEM FOR WOMEN AND MEN: THE EMERGING SCIENCE

## Epigenetics – the science behind the decline

For a long time, the scientific understanding of genetics took a limited outlook on our capacity for health and reproductive function. The theory had us believing your genes are your genes are your genes –

you are the product of your inheritance and there's not much you can do about it. However, it appears this is far from true. Over the past 10 – 20 years or so, scientists have become obsessed with the growing understanding of the field of epigenetics – an exciting field for us as it is continually demonstrating the benefits of the changes we can individually make to our genetic expression and overall health with our daily choices.

To understand the importance of epigenetics on fertility (specifically egg and sperm health), we need a little basic understanding of cellular reproduction. Our genes or genome refers to the strands of DNA that hold our blueprint for life, made up of the DNA from our biological parents – from their eggs and sperm. DNA basically controls the process of all our cells and their function. What we now realise is that changes in the conditions the cell is developing in and what the DNA is exposed to, can change which part of the gene is expressed (switched on or off), and therefore modify its development and function. This is called epigenetics – the ability for the expression of the gene to change depending on environment, without any change to the genetic code.

For a sense of your epigenetic potential, think about caterpillars turning into butterflies – while it has the same genetic DNA code, the expression of that code is fundamentally different through different stages in the lifecycle. DNA expression also depends on the environmental factors it was exposed to in the intracellular environment. If conditions are not right, the caterpillar will not become the butterfly. When it lives to its healthiest natural expression, it emerges from the cocoon with beautiful wings ready to fly.

Epigenetic scientists are now looking intently at how our lifestyle choices impact on how our inherited genetic factors play out. There is now much research to suggest genetic expression is highly influenced by three things:

1. What we ingest and absorb (what we eat and drink, the quality of the air we breathe and toxins we are exposed to like BPAs in plastics, man-made chemicals in our cleaning and personal products).

2. What we experience (stress and trauma).

3. How long we live (our age).

Sounds a lot like what we talk about with pre-conception care, doesn't it?

To ensure healthy DNA expression in all our cells as well as our eggs and sperm involves taking positive steps to avoid exposure in your lifestyle and diet. Eating and taking individually prescribed amounts of nutrients that support healthy expression of your DNA is critical to reduce the negative impacts as well, especially as we advance in years.

Epigenetics means 'above the genes' as it is a process called methylation that alters the way the genes are expressed. Methylation requires a number of nutrients to function appropriately, switching on and off the right gene expression at the right time. The quality of our DNA and its integrity, the energy our cells have for reproduction and the amount of oxidative stress our bodies are under all play a crucial role in the ageing of our bodies and our reproductive cells.

## Telomeres – the long and short of it.

One of the major barriers to healthy conception for women in their late 30s and 40s are the changes that occur, over time, to the DNA in all our cells including our eggs. Why? The rapidly evolving science of cellular aging is helping to give us some new indications about what is going on at the cellular level. At the end of our chromosomes (the strands of DNA) are sections called telomeres. Like the little plastic caps at the end of shoelaces that prevent our laces from unravelling, telomeres give stability to our DNA, preventing the strands from unravelling and helping them to connect properly when required for reproduction of cells. The longer these caps are, the more effective they are.

With age it seems our telomeres become shorter and shorter and science is beginning to understand this as a marker for health and cellular aging. The shorter our telomeres, the more likely we are to suffer chronic health conditions, including fertility problems.

---

### Health and fertility problems associated with short telomeres

o Infertility.[188,189]
o Chromosomal birth defects (Down Syndrome is commonly known but there are many more).[190]
o Miscarriage.[191]
o During pregnancy: pre-eclampsia.[192]
o Placental insufficiency.[193]
o Growth retardation in babies.[194]
o Type 2 diabetes.[194]
o Cardiovascular disease.[194]
o Liver disorders.[194]
o Various cancers.[195]
o Death from all causes.[196]

---

It seems no co-incidence that these are some of the more commonly-known risks for women who are trying to conceive at a later age. Conversely, conservation of telomere length parallels with exceptional longevity and health into older age and correlates with reproductive longevity. Nourishing healthy intact DNA in eggs and sperm is crucial as we age, as it is disruption to the DNA that causes chromosomal birth defects that are more commonly seen with older women and men trying to conceive. While in the infancy of research, it seems that common mechanism may underlie both, and the developing theories are gaining traction in the world of science.

## Apart from age, what else can shorten telomeres?

Along with genetic predisposition, telomeres are shortened over time by oxidative stress and genotoxic insults. Basically (and one reason why we are so excited about this theory) it turns out most of the things we suggest you avoid during preconception care will shorten your telomeres! Things like cigarette smoking, obesity, pesticides and herbicides in non-organic food, eating packaged and processed foods high in sugar and fat, man-made chemicals and heavy-metal exposure and stress or unhappiness all contribute to shorter telomeres.

The good news is that science is also emerging to support the theory that we can indeed improve the length of our telomeres! Our healthy recommendations are already in line with the research. A recent study showed for the first time that we can increase their length by making changes to our lifestyle at any age.[197] In this research, the greater the changes made, the longer the telomeres became.

Even more recent important research has shown that adopting regular yoga and meditation has a role in delaying/reversing aging and increasing quality of life in couples with unexplained infertility. The study suggests that these changes may increase the chance of natural conception and a healthy next generation by improving gamete structure and function.[198]

## How to increase your telomere length:[197-198]

- Follow a whole-food, low-fat, plant-based diet.
- Exercise regularly.
- Make stress-reduction techniques such as yoga and meditation a regular part of your life.
- And more social support – love and intimacy make for improvement in telomeres!

# Mito what? Mitochondria

These are the little organs within our cells that act as the powerhouse for all cellular function. Being the largest cell in the body, eggs rely on the mitochondria for their high-energy demands to replicate and divide. Sperm require healthy and abundant mitochondria to activate their tails and swim in the right direction. We have known for a long time that these mitochondrial organelles reduce in number and function as we age. With less energy-generating potential, the egg and any embryo resulting from conception cannot divide properly, leading to increased likelihood of chromosomal abnormalities, miscarriage and birth defects.

The DNA of mitochondria is also subjected to oxidative stress and these organelles unfortunately seem more susceptible than other parts of the cell.

> While reproductive science is working on methods for mitochondrial transplants, you can work on improving and stimulating the function of the existing mitochondria by reducing the load of damage causing oxidative stress with the recommended improvements to your diet and lifestyle, and increasing the nutrients required for protection and proper functioning of the energy cycle inside (more on this below). Some research has also suggested that exercise can increase the number of mitochondria.[199]

# Oxidative Stress – one of the biggest causes compromising healthy DNA

Oxidative stress and Reactive Oxygen Species (ROS) are a natural by-product of our metabolism but these unpaired electrons in our cells are highly reactive and can cause damage. As well as following our lifestyle recommendations to reduce any extra burden of ROS on our DNA and telomeres, a focus on antioxidants in your diet and supplementation regime is also super important for reducing the negative impacts in every cell – including your eggs and sperm.

## How to reduce oxidative stress

Antioxidants help to protect the developing eggs from damage to the DNA and the subsequent impact on our chance of conceiving and carrying a baby to full term. Antioxidants such as selenium, vitamin E, vitamin C, zinc, lipoic acid and coenzyme Q10 (CoQ10), appropriately and individually prescribed, are especially important for protecting the developing follicle and egg.

There is evidence to suggest that men may benefit by taking antioxidant supplements and increasing omega-3 fatty acids from fish and nuts.[200]

Eat foods containing antioxidants (selenium, vitamin E, vitamin C, zinc, CoQ10) at every meal every day, including fresh or frozen berries and brightly-coloured fruits and vegetables.

Sufficient therapeutic levels of antioxidants are important for many aspects of reproduction, but the importance of this supplementation grows with age. Please always consult with an expert in nutritional supplementation and fertility such as a naturopath for guidance with correct dosage for the most effective outcome in your particular case.

# Healthy cell division

Methylation is another important part of the process for producing healthy DNA, gene expression and hormone regulation, especially via epigenetics as we discussed above. You may not know it, but you likely (at least hopefully) are already taking a supplement to support methylation and a healthy pregnancy, as optimal methylation requires folate. Folate is the naturally-occurring form of this vitamin (vitamin B9) found in our foods. Metabolism of folate relies on a series of conversion steps as well as a number of enzyme activities before it can be used by our cells. Other vitamins such as B6 and B12 are also needed for this important methylation function.

It is thought that around 40 per cent of the population may have an inherited genetic alteration that impacts on our folate metabolism (MTHFR gene mutation – Methylenetetrahydrofolate reductase). Whilst it may affect a large percentage of the population and is relevant for both men and women, it may only be an issue for some. Other variables such as your B12 status and your homocysteine levels impact the effect it may have or supplementation required too. It is worthwhile discussing with your doctor or your naturopath whether these are tests you should consider, especially if you are older or have experienced:

o   Miscarriage.

o   Previous pregnancies with chromosomal abnormalities.

o   Any family history of chromosomal abnormalities.

o   Difficulty conceiving.[201,202]

It is a complex issue beyond the scope of this book, so we recommend you do seek the help of a qualified naturopath with fertility experience to ensure you get adequate exploration and support.

# IS EGG QUALITY AFFECTED BY OUR HORMONES?

If you have never done any work on balancing, regulating or improving your hormonal cycle, this can be life changing! The minor and sometimes more major symptoms of hormone imbalance can include irregular cycles, painful, heavy or very light periods, pre-menstrual tension, mood changes, excess hair growth, poor libido, hot flushes or night sweats, chocolate and sugar cravings, pimples, fluid retention … the list goes on! And you don't have to suffer!

Aside from a better quality of life, balancing the symphony of hormones required for ovulation to occur is fundamental for healthy egg development. It is so important to get all the basics right for your body's hormones to activate in the right amounts at the right time. Your body wants to be in balance and given the right materials (a healthy diet and lifestyle), healthy processing of used hormones (detoxification), avoidance of hormonal disruptors (chemicals such as BPA and phthalates in plastics or cosmetics) and a healthy attitude to stress, your body will respond accordingly and work towards attaining the right balance. Homoeostasis is the ultimate goal for all systems in the body under the right circumstances.

# WHAT IF I'M CONCERNED ABOUT MENOPAUSE?

If you are noticing signs of peri-menopause (the approach of menopause) such as irregular cycles, heavy periods, hot flushes or night sweats, a shorter than usual temper fuse, it is important to get to a GP or fertility specialist for thorough investigation. There are blood tests that can give you a clearer indication of your fertile potential and though not definitive they can certainly give you a good sense of how urgent your situation is. A full reproductive hormone profile on Day 2 or 3 of your cycle along with a progesterone test at Day 21 (or seven days after your ovulation) will be very helpful. Combined with an AMH (Anti Mullerian Hormone) test and someone knowledgeable to help with interpretation, you will get some sense of how impending menopause may be for you. Working with a fertility specialist to consider your options is a good idea; combined with collaborative practitioners in natural medicine, and applying all of our recommendations in this book will help you achieve the best outcome.

## SO WHAT ABOUT MEN'S AGEING AND FERTILITY?

It is true to say there has been far less investigation into the effects of ageing on fertility for men, however they don't escape the equation as we know sperm provide half of the genetic material for your baby and the healthier and more vital these cells, the healthier your pregnancy and baby is likely to be. It stands to reason that a vibrant, strong and resilient man has a greater chance of being a fabulous dad and his children's bodies and minds will reflect the lifestyle choices he is making before his partner conceives.

While some recent research has shown that exposure to polycyclic aromatic hydrocarbons (plastics, pesticides, dyes, burning wood or coal and smoking) will in fact shorten telomeres in sperm and compromise fertility[203], it appears that telomeres (see above) in fact lengthen in sperm as men age – a possible built-in evolutionary mechanism to improve the DNA of children conceived to older women. This doesn't let men off the hook though, as telomeres in most other cells are still shortening with age, leaving them susceptible to other chronic health conditions that increase inflammation and oxidative stress – a recipe for poor sperm development.

Due to their rapid turnover, thin outer membrane and smaller size, sperm are even more susceptible to oxidative stress and reduction in numbers and function of mitochondria as well. Similar theories in terms of DNA integrity and function apply here too. Adequate mitochondrial function is particularly important for sperm, as massive amounts of energy is required to drive the tail of the sperm, essential for the motility required to go the distance to reach the egg.

Virility, potency and stamina are also often noticeably reduced with age, so particular attention needs to be given to sexual function to ensure the sperm can get to where they need to go to meet the egg at just the right time of the reproductive cycle. Sometimes the added pressure of trying to conceive (especially if it has taken longer than you expected or been more difficult that you thought) can also be an issue for men. Wherever possible, it is important to address all the factors to improve fertility.

## HOW CAN WE IMPROVE EGG AND SPERM QUALITY?

Follow all the recommendations in our book! Do as much as you can and do it properly! You don't have any time to waste and you need to know you have done everything you can to give it your best shot.

## GIVE YOUR MITOCHONDRIA A BOOST

**Coenzyme Q10** is a powerful antioxidant and one of the key nutrients driving the energy production of the mitochondria. The developing egg has a high density of mitochondrial cells and so has a high requirement for coenzyme Q10. Our body makes CoQ10 (as well as getting some from animal foods) and it is thought this ability to make CoQ10 declines as we age. It follows that for optimal cellular health and egg and sperm quality, adequate levels of this substance is required.

CoQ10 (also known as ubiquinone) comes in many forms when taken as a supplement and not all are equal when it comes to the way your body absorbs and utilises it in the cells. Self-prescribing, especially the cheapest brands, is very likely to be a waste of time and money, so make sure you seek advice on this one.

When time is of the essence and age is a factor, we suggest supplementing with CoQ10; however, dietary sources include: seafood (mackerel), organ meats (only ever have organic), beef, pork, chicken, broccoli, parsley, oranges.

Other nutrients that are important for mitochondrial function include many of the B vitamins, Vitamin D, Vitamin C, E, alpha lipoic acid, acetyl-L-carnitine, N-acetyl cysteine, calcium, magnesium, selenium and essential fatty acids.

## INCREASE YOUR TELOMERES

**Essential fats** are essential for healthy cellular and mitochondrial membrane function and reducing any inflammation that may contribute to shortened telomeres! Ensure you are getting regular amounts of oily fish, avocado, nuts and seeds and cold-pressed extra virgin oils in your diet.

## GIVE YOUR DNA THE BEST CHANCE POSSIBLE

**Green leafy vegetables** give loads of folate required for methylation and healthy DNA. Even if you haven't been tested for the MTHFR gene mutation you can still ensure you up your folate levels by eating one to two cups of green leafy veggies daily such as spinach, asparagus, broccoli – plus include in your diet avocado, eggs, green peas, dried beans such as chickpeas and lentils. Folate supplementation is essential for everyone trying to conceive, ideal for at least three months prior to conception until you birth your baby. Ensure you are taking a minimum (across all supplements) of 400mcg/day. If you are over 35 or if you have been diagnosed with the MTHFR gene mutation, the requirements are higher, and supplements are available that are more readily utilised by people with this condition. In addition, as folate is a B vitamin it requires all the other B vitamins to be utilised properly by the body.

Methylation also depends on other nutrients including methionine and choline (found in protein foods), vitamin B6 (wholegrains, vegetables, nuts and meat) and B12 (meat, organic liver, shellfish and milk).

> As usual we recommend seeking advice from a naturopath about good levels of these nutrients suitable for you. There are many specific nutrients, herbs and other natural medicine supplements that have the potential to turn your fertility around. Of course, these are best individually assessed as specific nutrients come in different forms, the dose and quality of the supplement along with the length of time you need to be on these does vary significantly from person to person. Don't wast your time and money self prescribing – you will need expert advice on what you require for your specific needs.

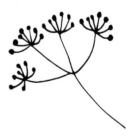

# Improve your blood flow to your eggs/sperm

Blood flow to your reproductive area is most important quite simply because this is how nourishing oxygen and nutrients are delivered to your eggs, and damaging wastes and toxins are carried away.

Exercise is so helpful. To move your blood around the ovarian area, focus on movement and exercise that moves your pelvis, abdominal area and legs. Walking and playing sports are great but have you thought of something outside of the obvious like belly-dancing or Latin dance? Both are excellent for getting your hips swinging and are known as sexy fertility dances for more than just how they look! It really does get the blood flowing! Kundalini or fertility yoga is also worth trying if you like to do yoga, and Pilates generally has a good focus on the pelvic and abdominal area as well. Or pick up a hula hoop and do a few minutes every day!

A cup or two of ginger tea will get your blood flowing! Simply slice up about a teaspoon of fresh ginger and let it soak in hot water for about five minutes before drinking. Add a little lemon if you like.

Hydration is of key importance for good healthy blood flow. Make sure you are drinking around eight glasses of filtered water a day.

Increased blood flow to the reproductive area is one of the many benefits of regular acupuncture treatment for your preconception period and whilst you are trying to conceive.

# HOW DO I KNOW WHEN
# I NEED EXTRA SUPPORT?

Seek extra support if you:

o   Are over 35.

o   Have a history or family history of miscarriage or a chromosomally abnormal pregnancy.

o   If you have already been trying to conceive for over six months.

o   Started menstruating before the age of 11 or after 16

o   Have ever had surgery on the ovaries such as endometriosis or PCOS

o   Have a history of smoking

o   Have a family history of early or premature menopause – ask your mum if she stopped menstruating before the age of 45.

Please ensure that any practitioner you see is an expert in working with fertility, and that they are open to collaborating with other practitioners such as naturopaths, Chinese medicine and medical doctors or fertility specialists. You never know when you need a team working with you for your best outcomes, so if you set it up from the beginning, you know you will get the best care for the longer term – and for your pregnancy, birthing environment and future family health.

If conceiving is taking longer than you thought or you are coming up against difficulties, we really encourage you to reach out for extra support with counselling, psychology or some kind of emotional-health consultation that works for you (you may consider kinesiology, life coaching, pastoral care or even find a support group to meet with). The possibilities for support are many and varied as there are many couples in the same position as you.

When it comes to the recommendations in this book and from your natural health team, we say just do it! You will feel better for it at all levels with more energy and vitality than you may have felt for years! It's is so good to know that you are giving it your best shot as you implement as many changes as is realistic for you, improving the health of all your cells, right down to your telomeres! And if you think you need motivation to achieve this end, what could be better than knowing this will give you the best chances of conceiving your healthy baby.

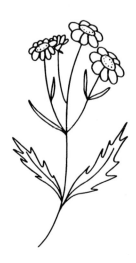

# TOP TIPS FOR HER

While women are born with all their eggs, a small portion of eggs undergo a maturation process in the lead up to each ovulation. During this time your eggs will be exposed to all the beneficial or harmful things you include in your life, so this is your opportunity to influence the health and to an extent, the age, of your eggs.

If you are over 35 you need to get cracking. All these things are relevant. Your age needs to be your motivator.

While you may feel you don't have time to make these changes, the point is that these approaches are designed to buy you time. Health is as important, if not more so, than time.

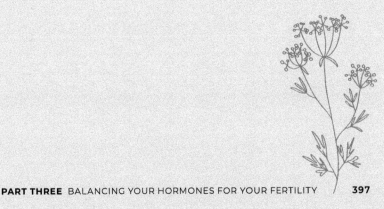

# TOP TIPS FOR HIM

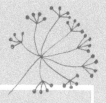

Sperm ages too, impacting the DNA, healthy conception and chances of having a healthy baby.

You are generating sperm right now that may be carrying the DNA that contributes to the formation of your baby. What you include and exclude from your diet and lifestyle in the three months prior to conceiving is of paramount importance as your developing sperm are exposed to everything you consume.

If you are already doing IVF don't just rely on ICSI. It is not a foolproof way to overcome the consequence of sperm defects most common in older men. The best of a bad lot may not actually be that good and still have all the negative effects we have outlined above.

# TOP TIPS FOR HIM AND HER

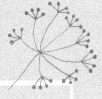

Eat one to two cups of green leafy vegies daily.

Increase your intake of antioxidants and essential fatty acids in your diet. Eat more oily fish, nuts, seeds and brightly-coloured fruit and vegetables.

Seek help from a professional for a tailored supplementation program specific for your requirements.

Exercise regularly and include stress reduction techniques on a regular basis.

Turn to the chapter on environmental factors affecting fertility in Chapter 7 for tips on improving egg and sperm quality.

Follow all of the recommendations in our book! Do as much as you can and start now. You don't have any time to waste and you need to know you have done everything you can to give it your best shot.

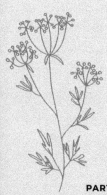

"YOU WILL GET THERE
WHEN YOU ARE MEANT
TO GET THERE AND NOT
ONE MOMENT SOONER ...
SO RELAX, BREATHE,
AND BE PATIENT"

MANDY HALE

APPENDIX 1

# Fertility boosting
## diet meal ideas

# SAMPLE DAILY DIET

## Breakfast

o   Oat, rice or quinoa porridge with pear or berries, LSA (grind up equal parts of linseeds, sunflower seeds and almonds) and natural yoghurt or soy milk and cinnamon powder.

o   Fruit-free muesli with natural yoghurt and grated apple.

o   Yogurt with berries and nuts.

o   Breakfast smoothie with a handful of greens like lettuce, spinach, rocket, avocado, chia seeds, milk of your choice, and blueberries.

o   Scrambled tofu/eggs with garlic mushrooms and roasted tomatoes.

o   Poached eggs with wilted spinach on seeded-bread toast.

o   Homemade baked beans with eggs, spinach, sheep milk/yoghurt/ cheese, parsley, avocado, whatever you like).

o   Omelette with goat's cheese, spring onions and left-over roast pumpkin.

o   Bone broth (chicken or beef) or miso soup with one to two eggs poached in it.

o   Bread or toast (sourdough, sprouted breads like Ezekiel, paleo bread, gluten free, nut and seed breads etc.) with:

   – *hummus and tomato.*

   – *sardines and a sprinkle of salt.*

   – *goats cheese and blueberries or poached fruit or sliced summer fruit (trust us!).*

   – *avocado and rocket.*

   – *black sesame paste and chopped fresh herbs like coriander and dill.*

o   Stew or bake fruit (apples, pears, quinces, rhubarb, berries ...) in
    a little water, grated ginger and cinnamon. Top cooked fruit with:

    – *lightly toasted chopped nuts (almond, walnut, pecan, Brazil, any!).*

    – *mix flaked dry coconut with LSA, buckwheat, chopped nuts,
       quinoa flakes ... your choice.*

    – *yoghurt (cow, sheep, goat, coconut etc).*

    – *ricotta.*

o   Miso soup with buckwheat noodles, tofu and vegetables.

## Lunch/dinner options

o   Grilled oily fish like salmon or sardines with fresh lemon/lime juice
    and freshly ground pepper with steamed vegetables and jacket
    baked sweet potato.

o   Stir fry tofu/chicken/lamb/beef with vegetables and brown rice.

o   Salad – mix it up by adding new ingredients:

    – *trout/sardines/salmon/chicken breast/lamb/beef.*

    – *boiled eggs.*

    – *marinated tofu or tempeh squares.*

    – *goat's cheese and roasted pumpkin.*

    – *dry fry seeds and nuts or add LSA or a sprinkle of sesame seeds.*

    – *beans/lentils/chickpeas.*

    – *falafel.*

    – *cooked quinoa or brown rice.*

    – *chopped fresh herbs like coriander, dill and/or parsley.*

    – *a lemon juice, olive oil, parsley and pepper dressing or yoghurt,
       mint and smoked paprika (avoid commercial dressings).*

- Rice cakes with salmon/fresh tomato/avocado/hummus.
- Soup: vegetables with lentils/beans/chickpeas/chicken, Asian-style broth with tofu/chicken, Miso soup with tofu and vegetables.
- Steamed chicken breast with mixed vegetables.
- Stir-fry-vegetables and tofu/tempeh/chicken with brown rice, tamari, garlic and ginger.
- Quinoa with roasted vegetables, cashew nuts and a yoghurt, tahini, lemon, honey and parsley sauce.
- Baked fish with roasted Mediterranean vegetables and olives or cherry tomatoes and rocket salad.
- Curries: vegetable curry/chicken/lamb/beef curry/fish curry/ dahl/chickpea curry with brown rice quinoa or cous cous and pappadums.
- Frittata with salad.

## Snacks

- Hummus, beetroot/eggplant/white bean /sweet potato dips (homemade best if you can due to poor quality oils in supermarket brands) or goat cheese with rice thins/wholegrain rice crackers/ vegetable sticks like cucumber, beans, carrot, celery, asparagus.
- Nuts and seeds: raw or lightly roasted with tamari and sesame oil.
- Rice thins or pappadams with avocado/sardines/hummus/tomato.
- Instant organic miso soup with tofu cubes.
- Natural yoghurt with organic berries and LSA.
- Kale chips (delicious and easily made by baking in the oven with a little olive oil, lemon juice and salt or try adding some spices and nutritional yeast flakes).

- Chickpeas: drain a BPA-free tin, rinse and toss in olive oil and spices and bake until crisp. Also makes a delicious addition to soup or salad as a crouton.

- Green smoothie: handful of greens, one banana or half cup of berries, teaspoon of nut butter, cup of water or coconut water, optional ¼ avocado for extra creaminess. Blend on high until smooth.

- Banana smoothie made with soy milk and LSA.

- Roasted veggies, olives, pine nuts and fetta wrapped in a lettuce leaf.

- Organic fresh or frozen berries (blueberries, cranberries, blackberries, raspberries, with nuts and seeds.

- Quality sugar-free peanut butter on slices of tomato with a little sea salt – seriously so good, try it!

- Slices of apple with tahini or any nut butter and cinnamon sprinkled on top.

## Drinks

- Water!

- Water with fruit or herbs soaked in it for flavor – any citrus slices, strawberries, cucumber, mint... let your imagination run wild!

- Mineral water with a squeeze of lemon/lime.

- Fresh vegetable juices.

- Herbal teas, hot or cold.

- Dandelion root tea.

- Spirulina, barley grass or chlorella added to water daily.

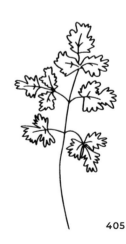

# Charting
your cycle

Download this chart from our website to print out in full A4 size and use at home – *www.bit.ly/fertilitychart*

# REPRODUCTIVE CYCLE CHART

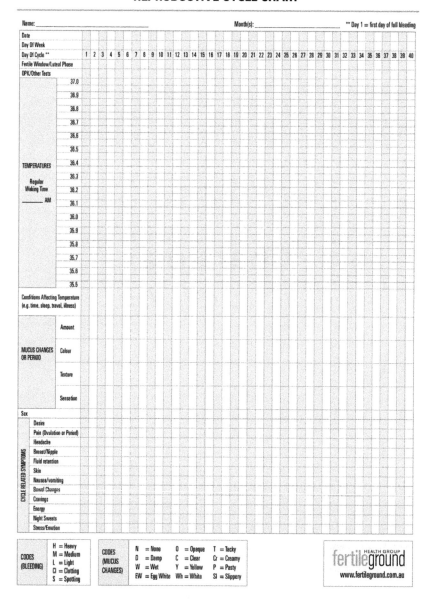

CREATE A FERTILE LIFE

# CHARTING INSTRUCTIONS FOR CONSCIOUS CONCEPTION

Where time permits, it is useful to check and record the signs and symptoms of your reproductive cycle for a few cycles before you try to conceive. Knowing your signs of ovulation and timing your sex with understanding of your cycle will give you an increased sense of confidence in your conscious conception. Marking secondary symptoms like headaches or fluid retention will give very useful information about your cycle and hormones to assist with providing the best treatment for your individual needs.

# CHECKING AND RECORDING YOUR CERVICAL MUCUS CHANGES

o   Check your mucus each time you go to the toilet (before urination). For a more accurate way to track your mucus; insert your finger 1-2 cm into the vaginal entrance, then remove your finger. Stretch out any mucus between that finger and your thumb. Record the amount, colour, texture, and external sensation on your chart. Always record the most fertile mucus you noticed that day.

o   Your basic infertile pattern of mucus can vary from none/dry or damp, pasty, flaky, crumbly, thick, dense in the non-fertile phases. As ovulation approaches, the mucus pattern will change to creamy or milky and start to increase and become wetter. Your fertile mucus will be clear, wet, watery, slimy, slippery or stretchy at ovulation, more like raw egg white.

o   How does the outside of your vagina feel? Is it wet or dry, moist or damp? Is there a lot of it, a medium amount or very little. The wetter the sensation, the more fertile you are.

- You are most fertile in the two days before and on the day of ovulation. This is your Fertile Window. This clear, egg white mucus will help the sperm to reach the egg.

- Immediately after ovulation, there is a marked decrease in mucus production, with a quick return to your basic infertile pattern. You can confirm ovulation has occurred if you are charting your temperature as well (see below).

## CHECKING AND RECORDING YOUR RESTING TEMPERATURE

- You need a digital thermometer designed for under-the-tongue use (not an ear thermometer).

- Have the thermometer beside your bed before you go to sleep. On waking, before getting out of bed or even talking, take your temperature by placing the thermometer under your tongue. It is important to make as little movement as possible whilst taking your temperature to get a true resting temperature. On your chart place a dot in the box that corresponds to your temperature and day of cycle.

- Many thermometers keep the temperature displayed until you use it again, so you don't have to record it straight away if it is still dark or you are trying not to wake your partner.

- Your temperature needs to be taken ideally at the same time each morning after at least 5 hours consecutive sleep. Mark your regular waking time, and record any variation. When you sleep in, record the temperature and add a second mark 0.05 down (one box) for every 1/2 hour extra sleep. If you wake up early, adjust your temperature 0.05 up for every 1/2 hour.

- Usually, there will be a "thermal shift" of about 1/2 a degree Celsius that indicates ovulation has occurred. The temperature starts to shift after the egg is released. The rule is 3 over 5 – you need to see three mornings of higher temperatures than the last five. This is why you can't use temperature charts to time your conception attempts, as once the shift has occurred, ovulation is already over and you have missed your chance. You can however record any sex you have had and use your chart to see if you did indeed get the timing right in that cycle to know that you are in with a chance.

- Conditions that may affect your temperature may include things like a late night, fever, a cold, sleeping in, broken sleep or alcohol. These may cause abnormally high or low temperatures, so it is important to record them for understanding your temperatures when looking back over time.

## MAKING SENSE OF IT

If you want to understand more about your hormones and charting your cycle find a fertility naturopath. Scan and email or bring your charts to every appointment where possible. Your practitioner will help you to understand and interpret your chart with ease. It may seem confusing at first, but within a few cycles, it will become clear - a free and easy method to understand your cycle for your reproductive life.

# What to do next if you're looking for more help

Check us out (the authors) if you're looking for more support. Fertile Ground Health Group is a leading natural medicine fertility clinic in Melbourne. We have some of the most experienced practitioners in the treatment of fertility, pregnancy and family health. We are committed to providing expert care and compassionate support to help patients achieve their families.

Expert services include naturopathic fertility treatment, acupuncture and Chinese herbal medicine, IVF support, obstetrics and gynecology, pregnancy massage, osteopathy for mothers and babies, counselling and birth attendants/doulas.

For naturopathic fertility consultations in person in Melbourne or online for anywhere else in the world, contact Fertile Ground Health Group and book in for a consultation with Gina Fox, Rhiannon Hardingham , Tina Jenkins or anyone on our expert team. Acupuncture and Chinese herbal medicine, obstetrics and gynecology, osteopathy, massage, counselling and birth attendants are also available with some of Australia's best practitioners.

Book online *www.fertileground.com.au*
or call the clinic +61 (3) 9419 9988

For Charmaine and Gina's guided relaxations specifically for natural conception, IVF and pregnancy download from *www.befertile.com.au* or go to iTunes and search Be Fertile.

For informed writing, blogs, podcasts and our online shop, check out our website *www.fertileground.com.au*, like us on Facebook *www.facebook.com/fertilegroundhealthgroup* and follow our Instagram page *www.instagram.com/fertile_ground_health_group/*

For inspiring podcasts on fertility topics by Fertile Ground practitioners Gina Fox and Jo Sharkey go to your podcast app or iTunes and search for Finding Fertility podcast. *www.findingfertilitypodcast.com*

We are also fertility health educators and speak on a range of fertility related topics. For speakers, practitioner mentoring sessions or masterclass sign up, contact naturopaths Rhiannon Hardingham, Charmaine Dennis and Gina Fox at Fertile Ground Health Group. Email: *management@fertileground.com.au*

For health practitioner business mentoring and revitalise your business local workshops or overseas retreats, contact Charmaine Dennis at *management@fertileground.com.au*

## Further reading

Bijlsma, Nicole, *Healthy Home Healthy Family*, Australian College of Environmental Studies, 2018

Cabrall, Josephine, *The PCOS Solution: An evidence-based naturopathic guide to clear skin, regular periods and fertility*, My Vagina Pty Ltd, 2017

Dempsey, Rhea, *Birthing Wisdom*, Boathouse Press, 2013

Fett, Rebecca, *It Starts with the Egg*, Franklin Fox Publishing, New York, 2014

Fertility Coalition public education program Your Fertility *www.yourfertility.org.au*

Jennings, Tasha , *The Fertility Diet*, Wilkinson Publishing, 2015

Joly, Petra, *The Fertility Food Map*, Newtown Natural Fertilty, 2017

Kirkpatrick, Belinda & Johnstone, Ainsley, *Healthy Hormones: A Practical Guide to Balancing your hormones*, Murdoch Books Australia, 2018

Kringoudis, Nat, *Well & Good: Supercharge Your Health For Fertility & Wellness*, Melbourne University Press, 2014

McIntosh, Tabitha & Lantz, Sarah, *One Bite at a Time*, 2016

Naish, Francesca, *Natural Fertility*, Sarah Milner Publishing, 2000

Tricky, Ruth, *Women, Hormones & the Menstrual Cycle*, Trickey Enterprises (Victoria) Pty Limited, 2011

Safer skin care products *www.ewg.org/skindeep*

The Chemical Maze
*www.chemicalmaze.com*

Consult the Environmental working group guide to sunscreens at *www.ewg.org/2015sunscreen/*

WHO endocrine disrupters
*www.who.int/ceh/risks/cehemerging2/en/*

'Shoppers Guide to Pesticides in Produce™' by the Environmental Working Group at *www.ewg.org.*

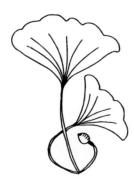

# References

1.    Fritz MA, Speroff L. *Clinical Gynecologic Endocrinology and Infertility.*
      8th edn. Philadelphia: Wolters Kluwer Health/Lippincott Williams
      & Wilkins; 2011.

2.    Thoma ME, McLain AC, Louis JF, et al. Prevalence of infertility in the
      United States as estimated by the current duration approach and
      a traditional constructed approach. *Fertil Steril.* 2013;99(5):1324-1331.
      doi:10.1016/j.fertnstert.2012.11.037.

3.    Loxton D, Lucke J. *Reproductive Health: Findings from the Australian
      Longitudinal Study on Women's Health.*; 2010. http://www.alswh.org.au/
      images/content/pdf/major_reports/2009_major_report_d_r149.pdf.

4.    Rai R, Regan L. Recurrent miscarriage. *Lancet.* 2006;368(9535):601-611.
      doi:10.1016/S0140-6736(06)69204-0.

5.    Levine H, Jørgensen N, Martino-Andrade A, et al. Temporal trends in
      sperm count: A systematic review and meta-regression analysis. *Hum
      Reprod Update.* 2017;23(6):646-659. doi:10.1093/humupd/dmx022.

6.    Ilacqua A, Izzo G, Emerenziani G Pietro, Baldari C, Aversa A. Lifestyle
      and fertility: The influence of stress and quality of life on male fertility.
      *Reprod Biol Endocrinol.* 2018;16(1):1-11. doi:10.1186/s12958-018-0436-9.

7.    Salas-Huetos A, Bulló M, Salas-Salvadó J. Dietary patterns, foods and
      nutrients in male fertility parameters and fecundability: A systematic
      review of observational studies. *Hum Reprod Update.* 2017;23(4):371-389.
      doi:10.1093/humupd/dmx006.

8.    Gaskins AJ, Chavarro JE. Diet and fertility: a review. *Am J Obstet Gynecol.*
      2018;218(4):379-389. doi:10.1016/j.ajog.2017.08.010.

9.    Hampton KD, Mazza D, Newton JM. Fertility-awareness knowledge,
      attitudes, and practices of women seeking fertility assistance. *J Adv Nurs.*
      2013;69(5):1076-1084. doi:10.1111/j.1365-2648.2012.06095.x.

10.   Cancer Council Vic. Cancer Council Victoria. Is your weight healthy?
      http://www.cancervic.org.au/preventing-cancer/weight/bmi.
      Accessed June 9, 2017.

11.   Morán C, Hernández E, Ruíz JE, Fonseca ME, Bermúdez JA, Zárate
      A. Upper body obesity and hyperinsulinemia are associated with
      anovulation. *Gynecol Obstet Invest.* 1999;47(1):1-5. doi:10.1159/000010052.

12.     Singh D. Female mate value at a glance: relationship of waist-to-hip ratio to health, fecundity and attractiveness. *Neuro Endocrinol Lett*. 2002;23 Suppl 4(December):81-91.

13.     Leisegang K, Bouic PJ, Menkveld R, Henkel RR. Obesity is associated with increased seminal insulin and leptin alongside reduced fertility parameters in a controlled male cohort. *Reprod Biol Endocrinol*. 2014;12(34):1780. doi:10.1016/j.juro.2014.09.073.

14.     Department of Health. *Australia's Physical Activity and Sedentary Behaviour Guidelines*. ACT, Australia: Commonwealth of Australia; 2014. http://www.health.gov.au/internet/main/publishing.nsf/content/health-pubhlth-strateg-phys-act-guidelines. Accessed June 7, 2017.

15.     Ried K. Chinese herbal medicine for female infertility : An updated meta-analysis. *Complement Ther Med*. 2015;23(1):116-128. doi:10.1016/j.ctim.2014.12.004.

16.     Tan L, Tong Y, Sze SCW, et al. Chinese Herbal Medicine for Infertility with Anovulation: A Systematic Review. *J Altern Complement Med*. 2012;18(12):1087-1100. doi:10.1089/acm.2011.0371.

17.     Johansson J, Redman L, Veldhuis PP, et al. Acupuncture for ovulation induction in polycystic ovary syndrome: a randomized controlled trial. *Am J Physiol Endocrinol Metab*. 2013;304(9):E934-43. doi:10.1152/ajpendo.00039.2013.

18.     Smith CA, Armour M, Shewamene Z, Tan HY, Norman RJ, Johnson NP. Acupuncture performed around the time of embryo transfer: a systematic review and meta-analysis. *Reprod Biomed Online*. 2019;00(0):1-16. doi:https://doi.org/10.1016/j.rbmo.2018.12.038.

19.     A SC, Mike A, Xiaoshu Z, Xun L, Yong LZ, Jing S. Acupuncture for dysmenorrhoea. *Cochrane Database Syst Rev*. 2016;(4). doi:10.1002/14651858.CD007854.pub3.

20.     Hullender Rubin LE, Opsahl MS, Wiemer K, Mist SD, Caughey AB, Hullender LE. Impact of Whole Systems Traditional Chinese Medicine on In Vitro Fertilization Outcomes HHS Public Access. *Reprod Biomed Online*. 2015;30(6):602-612. doi:10.1016/j.rbmo.2015.02.005.

21.     Chen Y, Fang Y, Yang J, Wang F, Wang Y, Yang L. Effect of acupuncture on premature ovarian failure: A pilot study. *Evidence-based Complement Altern Med*. 2014;2014:2-7. doi:10.1155/2014/718675.

22.     Manheimer E, Zhang G, Udoff L, et al. Effects of acupuncture on rates of pregnancy and live birth among women undergoing in vitro fertilisation: Systematic review and meta-analysis. *Bmj*. 2008;336(7643):545-549. doi:10.1136/bmj.39471.430451.BE.

23. Guo J, Wang L, Li D. [Exploring the effects of Chinese medicine in improving uterine endometrial blood flow for increasing the successful rate of in vitro fertilization and embryo transfer]. *Zhong Xi Yi Jie He Xue Bao*. 2011;9(12):1301-1306. http://www.ncbi.nlm.nih.gov/pubmed/22152767. Accessed February 8, 2019.

24. Habek D, Čerkez Habek J, Bobić-Vuković M, Vujić B. Efficacy of Acupuncture for the Treatment of Primary Dysmenorrhea. *Gynakol Geburtshilfliche Rundsch*. 2003;43(4):250-253. doi:10.1159/000072730.

25. Zijlstra FJ, Van Den Berg-De Lange I, Huygen FJPM, Klein J. Anti-inflammatory actions of acupuncture. *Mediators Inflamm*. 2003;12(2):59-69. doi:10.1080/0962935031000114943.

26. Sherman S, Eltes F, Wolfson V, Zabludovsky N, Bartoov B. Effect of acupuncture on sperm parameters of males suffering from subfertility related to low sperm quality. *Syst Biol Reprod Med*. 1997;39(2):155-161. doi:10.3109/01485019708987914.

27. Dong C, Chen S, Jiang J, et al. [Clinical observation and study of mechanisms of needle-picking therapy for primary infertility of abnormal sperm]. *Zhongguo Zhen Jiu*. 2006;26(6):389-391. http://www.ncbi.nlm.nih.gov/pubmed/16813177. Accessed August 5, 2018.

28. Balk J, Catov J, Horn B, Gecsi K, Wakim A. The relationship between perceived stress, acupuncture, and pregnancy rates among IVF patients: a pilot study. *Complement Ther Clin Pr*. 2010;16(3):154-157. doi:10.1111/j.1743-6109.2008.01122.x.Endothelial.

29. Isoyama D, Cordts EB, De Souza Van Niewegen AMB, De Almeida Pereira De Carvalho W, Matsumura ST, Barbosa CP. Effect of acupuncture on symptoms of anxiety in women undergoing in vitro fertilisation: A prospective randomised controlled study. *Acupunct Med*. 2012;30(2):85-88. doi:10.1136/acupmed-2011-010064.

30. Ulbricht C, Chao W, Costa D, Rusie-Seamon E, Weissner W, Woods J. Clinical evidence of herb-drug interactions: a systematic review by the natural standard research collaboration. *Curr Drug Metab*. 2008;9(10):1063-1120. http://www.ncbi.nlm.nih.gov/pubmed/19075623. Accessed March 8, 2019.

31. Sørensen JM. Herb–Drug, Food–Drug, Nutrient–Drug, and Drug–Drug Interactions: Mechanisms Involved and Their Medical Implications. *J Altern Complement Med*. 2002;8(3):293-308. doi:10.1089/10755530260127989.

32. de Boer A, van Hunsel F, Bast A. Adverse food-drug interactions. *Regul Toxicol Pharmacol*. 2015;73(3):859-865. doi:10.1016/j.yrtph.2015.10.009.

33. Cheong YC, Dix S, Hung Yu Ng E, Ledger WL, Farquhar C. Acupuncture and assisted reproductive technology. *Cochrane Database Syst Rev.* 2013;(7). doi:10.1002/14651858.CD006920.pub3.

34. Bouter LM, Manheimer E, Liu J, et al. The effects of acupuncture on rates of clinical pregnancy among women undergoing in vitro fertilization: a systematic review and meta-analysis. *Hum Reprod Update.* 2013;19(6):696-713. doi:10.1093/humupd/dmt026.

35. Shen C, Wu M, Shu D, Zhao X, Gao Y. The role of acupuncture in in vitro fertilization: A systematic review and meta-analysis. *Gynecol Obstet Invest.* 2015;79(1):1-12. doi:10.1159/000362231.

36. Zheng CH, Zhang MM, Huang GY, Wang W. The role of acupuncture in assisted reproductive technology. *Evidence-based Complement Altern Med.* 2012;2012. doi:10.1155/2012/543924.

37. Cao H, Han M, Ng EHY, et al. Can Chinese Herbal Medicine Improve Outcomes of In Vitro Fertilization? A Systematic Review and Meta-Analysis of Randomized Controlled Trials. *PLoS One.* 2013;8(12):e81650. doi:10.1371/journal.pone.0081650.

38. de Lacey S, Smith CA, Paterson C. Building resilience: A preliminary exploration of women's perceptions of the use of acupuncture as an adjunct to In Vitro Fertilisation. *BMC Complement Altern Med.* 2009;9:1-11. doi:10.1186/1472-6882-9-50.

39. Domar AD, Meshay I, Kelliher J, Alper M, Powers RD. The impact of acupuncture on in vitro fertilization outcome. *Fertil Steril.* 2009;91(3): 723-726. doi:10.1016/j.fertnstert.2008.01.018.

40. Smith CA, de Lacey S, Chapman M, et al. The effects of acupuncture on the secondary outcomes of anxiety and quality of life for women undergoing IVF: A randomized controlled trial. *Acta Obstet Gynecol Scand.* 2019;(October 2018):1-10. doi:10.1111/aogs.13528.

41. Jansen RPS. Elusive fertility: fecundability and assisted conception in perspective. *Fertil Steril.* 1995;64(2):252-254. doi:10.1016/S0015-0282(16)57718-8.

42. Gnoth C, Godehardt D, Godehardt E, Frank-Herrmann P, Freundl G. Time to pregnancy: Results of the German prospective study and impact on the management of infertility. *Hum Reprod.* 2003;18(9):1959-1966. doi:10.1093/humrep/deg366.

43. Te Velde ER, Eijkemans R, Habbema H. Variation in couple fecundity and time to pregnancy, an essential concept in human reproduction. *Lancet.* 2000;355(June):1928-1929. doi:10.1016/S0140-6736(00)03202-5.

44. Crosignani P, Rubin B, The ESHRE Capri Workshop Group. Optimal use of infertility diagnostic tests and treatments. *Hum Reprod.* 2000;15(3):723-732. doi:10.1093/humrep/15.3.723.

45. Sharma R, Biedenharn KR, Fedor JM, Agarwal A. Lifestyle factors and reproductive health: taking control of your fertility. *Reprod Biol Endocrinol.* 2013;11(1):66. doi:10.1186/1477-7827-11-66.

46. Manders M, McLindon L, Schulze B, Beckmann MM, Kremer JAM, Farquhar C. Timed intercourse for couples trying to conceive. *Cochrane database Syst Rev.* 2015;3(3):CD011345. doi:10.1002/14651858.CD011345.pub2.

47. Hampton K, Mazza D. Fertility-awareness knowledge, attitudes and practices of women attending general practice. *Aust Fam Physician.* 2015;44(11):840-845.

48. Evans-Hoeker E, Pritchard DA, Long DL, Herring AH, Stanford JB, Steiner AZ. Cervical mucus monitoring prevalence and associated fecundability in women trying to conceive. *Fertil Steril.* 2013;100(4):1033-1038.e1. doi:10.1016/j.fertnstert.2013.06.002.

49. Gosálvez J, González-Martínez M, López-Fernández C, Fernández JL, Sánchez-Martín P. Shorter abstinence decreases sperm deoxyribonucleic acid fragmentation in ejaculate. *Fertil Steril.* 2011;96(5):1083-1086. doi:10.1016/j.fertnstert.2011.08.027.

50. Pons I, Cercas R, Villas C, Braña C, Fernández-Shaw S. One abstinence day decreases sperm DNA fragmentation in 90 % of selected patients. *J Assist Reprod Genet.* 2013;30(9):1211-1218. doi:10.1007/s10815-013-0089-8.

51. Greening D. Frequent ejaculation. a pilot study of changes in sperm DNA damage and semen parameters using daily ejaculation. *Fertil Steril.* 2007;88(Supplement 1):S19-S20.

52. Practice Committee of the American Society for Reproductive Medicine in collaboration with the Society for Reproductive Endocrinology and Infertility. Optimizing natural fertility: a committee opinion. *Fertil Steril.* 2017;107(1):52-58. doi:10.1016/j.fertnstert.2016.09.029.

53. Tao P, Coates R, Maycock B. The impact of infertility on sexuality: A literature review. *Australas Med J.* 2011;4(11):620-627. doi:10.4066/AMJ.2011.1055.

54. Tremellen KP. The effect of intercourse on pregnancy rates during assisted human reproduction. *Hum Reprod.* 2000;15(12):2653-2658. doi:10.1093/humrep/15.12.2653.

55. Munafo M, Murphy M, Whiteman D, Hey K. Does cigarette smoking increase time to conception?. *J Biosoc Sci.* 2002;34(1):65-73. doi:10.1017/S0021932002000652.

56. Augood C, Duckitt K, Templeton a a. Smoking and female infertility: a systematic review and meta-analysis. *Hum Reprod*. 1998;13(6):1532-1539. doi:10.1093/humrep/13.6.1532.

57. Fertility Coalition. Smoking and fertility. Your Fertility Website. https://yourfertility.org.au/for-women/smoking-and-fertility/. Accessed August 5, 2018.

58. Depa-Martynów M, Jedrzejczak P, Taszarek-Hauke G, Jósiak M, Pawelczyk L. The impact of cigarette smoking on oocytes and embryos quality during in vitro fertilization program. *Przegląd Lek*. 2003;63(10):838-840.

59. Mendelsohn C, Gould G, Oncken C. Management of smoking in pregnant women. *Aust Fam Physician*. 2014;31(1):30-38.

60. Penzias A, Bendikson K, Butts S, et al. Smoking and infertility: a committee opinion. *Fertil Steril*. 2018;110(4):611-618. doi:10.1016/j.fertnstert.2018.06.016.

61. Shiloh H, LahavBaratz S, Koifman M, et al. The impact of cigarette smoking on zona pellucida thickness of oocytes and embryos prior to transfer into the uterine cavity. *Hum Reprod*. 2004;19(1):157-159. doi:10.1093/humrep/deh029.

62. Harlev A, Agarwal A, Gunes SO, Shetty A, du Plessis SS. Smoking and Male Infertility: An Evidence-Based Review. *World J Mens Health*. 2015;33(3):143. doi:10.5534/wjmh.2015.33.3.143.

63. Shiri R, Häkkinen J, Koskimäki J, Tammela TLJ, Auvinen A, Hakama M. Smoking causes erectile dysfunction through vascular disease. *Urology*. 2006;68(6):1318-1322. doi:10.1016/j.urology.2006.08.1088.

64. Vine MF, Tse CK, Hu P, Truong KY. Cigarette smoking and semen quality. *Fertil Steril*. 1996;65(4):835-842. doi:10.1016/S0015-0282(16)58223-5.

65. Selit I, Basha M, Maraee A, et al. Sperm DNA and RNA abnormalities in fertile and oligoasthenoteratozoospermic smokers. *Andrologia*. 2013;45(1):35-39. doi:10.1111/j.1439-0272.2012.01305.x.

66. Zitzmann M, Rolf C, Nordhoff V, et al. Male smokers have a decreased success rate for in vitro fertilization and intracytoplasmic sperm injection. *Fertil Steril*. 2003;79(SUPPL. 3):1550-1554. doi:10.1016/S0015-0282(03)00339-X.

67. Blanco-Munoz J, Torres-Sánchez L, López-Carrillo L. Exposure to maternal and paternal tobacco consumption and risk of spontaneous abortion. *Public Health Rep*. 2009;124(2):317-322. http://search.ebscohost.com/login.aspx?direct=true&db=jlh&AN=105452679&site=ehost-live.

68. Hull MGR, North K, Taylorb H, Farrow A, Christopher L Ford W. Delayed conception and active and passive smoking. *Fertil Steril*. 2000;74(4):725-733. doi:10.1016/S0015-0282(00)01501-6.

69.     Hyland A, Piazza KM, Hovey KM, et al. Associations of lifetime active and passive smoking with spontaneous abortion, stillbirth and tubal ectopic pregnancy: a cross-sectional analysis of historical data from the Women's Health Initiative. *Tob Control*. 2015;24(4):328-335. doi:10.1136/tobaccocontrol-2013-051458.

70.     Neuman Å, Hohmann C, Orsini N, et al. Maternal smoking in pregnancy and asthma in preschool children: A pooled analysis of eight birth cohorts. *Am J Respir Crit Care Med*. 2012;186(10):1037-1043. doi:10.1164/rccm.201203-0501OC.

71.     Hakeem GF, Oddy L, Holcroft CA, Abenhaim HA. Incidence and determinants of sudden infant death syndrome: a population-based study on 37 million births. *World J Pediatr*. 2014;11(1):41-47. doi:10.1007/s12519-014-0530-9.

72.     Hackshaw A, Rodeck C, Boniface S. Maternal smoking in pregnancy and birth defects: A systematic review based on 173 687 malformed cases and 11.7 million controls. *Hum Reprod Update*. 2011;17(5):589-604. doi:10.1093/humupd/dmr022.

73.     Heck JE, Contreras ZA, Park AS, Davidson TB, Cockburn M, Ritz B. Smoking in pregnancy and risk of cancer among young children: A population-based study. *Int J Cancer*. 2016;139(3):613-616. doi:10.1002/ijc.30111.

74.     Button TMM, Thapar A, McGuffin P. Relationship between antisocial behaviour, attention-deficit hyperactivity disorder and maternal prenatal smoking. *Br J Psychiatry*. 2005;187(AUG.):155-160. doi:10.1192/bjp.187.2.155.

75.     Buka SL, Shenassa ED, Niaura R. Elevated risk of tobacco dependence among offspring of mothers who smoked during pregnancy: A 30-year prospective study. *Am J Psychiatry*. 2003;160(11):1978-1984. doi:10.1176/appi.ajp.160.11.1978.

76.     Ekblad M, Gissler M, Lehtonen L, Korkeila J. Prenatal Smoking Exposure and the Risk of Psychiatric Morbidity Into Young Adulthood. *Arch Gen Psychiatry*. 2010;67(8):841. doi:10.1001/archgenpsychiatry.2010.92.

77.     Camlin NJ, Sobinoff AP, Sutherland JM, et al. Maternal Smoke Exposure Impairs the Long-Term Fertility of Female Offspring in a Murine Model1. *Biol Reprod*. 2016;94(2):1-12. doi:10.1095/biolreprod.115.135848.

78.     Sépaniak S, Forges T, Monnier-Barbarino P. Cigarette smoking and fertility in women and men. *Gynécologie Obs Fertil*. 2006;34(10):945-949. doi:10.1016/j.gyobfe.2006.06.018.

79.     Agency ANPH, Developer VM by T. Quit Now: My QuitBuddy. iTunes. https://itunes.apple.com/au/app/quit-now-my-quitbuddy/id527485761?mt=8. Published 2017. Accessed August 20, 2017.

80. NHMRC. Australian Guidelines to Reduce Health Risks from Drinking Alcohol. 2009. doi:10.1037/e509232012-001.

81. Gormack AA, Peek JC, Derraik JGB, Gluckman PD, Young NL, Cutfield WS. Many women undergoing fertility treatment make poor lifestyle choices that may affect treatment outcome. *Hum Reprod.* 2015;30(7):1617-1624. doi:10.1093/humrep/dev094.

82. Homan GF, Davies M, Norman R, G.F. H, M. D. The impact of lifestyle factors on reproductive performance in the general population and those undergoing infertility treatment: A review. *Hum Reprod Update.* 2007;13(3):209-223. doi:10.1093/humupd/dml056.

83. Kesmodel U, Wisborg K, Olsen SF, Henriksen TB, Secher NJ. Moderate alcohol intake in pregnancy and the risk of spontaneous abortion. *Alcohol Alcohol.* 2002;37(1):87-92. doi:10.1093/alcalc/37.1.87.

84. Condorelli RA, Calogero AE, Vicari E, La Vignera S. Chronic consumption of alcohol and sperm parameters: Our experience and the main evidences. *Andrologia.* 2015;47(4):368-379. doi:10.1111/and.12284.

85. Hatch EE, Bracken MB. Association of delayed conception with caffeine consumption. *Am J Epidemiol.* 1993;138(12):1082-1092. http://www.ncbi.nlm.nih.gov/pubmed/8266910. Accessed January 25, 2019.

86. Greenwood D, Thatcher N, Ye J, et al. Caffeine intake during pregnancy and adverse birth outcomes: a systematic review and dose-response meta-analysis. *Eur J Epidemiol.* 2014;29(10):725-734.

87. Louis GMB, Lum KJ, Sundaram R, et al. Window : Evidence in Support of Relaxation. 2012;95(7):2184-2189. doi:10.1016/j.fertnstert.2010.06.078.Stress.

88. Ricci E, Viganò P, Cipriani S, et al. Coffee and caffeine intake and male infertility: A systematic review. *Nutr J.* 2017;16(1):1-14. doi:10.1186/s12937-017-0257-2.

89. Braga DPDAF, Halpern G, Figueira RDCS, Setti AS, Iaconelli A, Borges E. Food intake and social habits in male patients and its relationship to intracytoplasmic sperm injection outcomes. *Fertil Steril.* 2012;97(1):53-59. doi:10.1016/j.fertnstert.2011.10.011.

90. Ulvik A, Vollset SE, Hoff G, Ueland PM. Coffee Consumption and Circulating B-Vitamins in Healthy Middle-Aged Men and Women. *Clin Chem.* 2008;54(9):1489-1496. doi:10.1373/clinchem.2008.103465.

91. Food Standards Australia New Zealand. Caffeine. http://www.foodstandards.gov.au/consumer/generalissues/Pages/Caffeine.aspx. Published 2018. Accessed August 5, 2018.

92. du Plessis SS, Agarwal A, Syriac A. Marijuana, phytocannabinoids, the endocannabinoid system, and male fertility. *J Assist Reprod Genet.* 2015;32(11):1575-1588. doi:10.1007/s10815-015-0553-8.

93.     Fronczak CM, Kim ED, Barqawi AB. The insults of illicit drug use on male fertility. *J Androl*. 2012;33(4):515-528. doi:10.2164/jandrol.110.011874.

94.     Brents LK. Marijuana, the endocannabinoid system and the female reproductive system. *Yale J Biol Med*. 2016;89(2):175-191.

95.     Klonoff-Cohen HS, Natarajan L, Victoria Chen R. A prospective study of the effects of female and male marijuana use on in vitro fertilization (IVF) and gamete intrafallopian transfer (GIFT) outcomes. *Am J Obstet Gynecol*. 2006;194(2):369-376. doi:10.1016/j.ajog.2005.08.020.

96.     Fergusson DM, Horwood LJ, Northstone K. Maternal use of cannabis and pregnancy outcome. *BJOG An Int J Obstet Gynaecol*. 2002;109(1):21-27. doi:10.1111/j.1471-0528.2002.01020.x.

97.     Pandey S, Pandey S, Maheshwari A, Bhattacharya S. The impact of female obesity on the outcome of fertility treatment. *J Hum Reprod Sci*. 2010;3(2):62-67. doi:10.4103/0974-1208.69332.

98.     Kort JD, Winget C, Kim SH, Lathi RB. A retrospective cohort study to evaluate the impact of meaningful weight loss on fertility outcomes in an overweight population with infertility. *Fertil Steril*. 2014;101(5):1400-1403. doi:10.1016/j.fertnstert.2014.01.036.

99.     Shayeb AG, Harrild K, Mathers E, Bhattacharya S. An exploration of the association between male body mass index and semen quality. *Reprod Biomed Online*. 2011;23(6):717-723. doi:10.1016/j.rbmo.2011.07.018.

100.    Hammoud AO, Gibson M, Peterson CM, Meikle AW, Carrell DT. Impact of male obesity on infertility: a critical review of the current literature. *Fertil Steril*. 2008;90(4):897-904. doi:10.1016/j.fertnstert.2008.08.026.

101.    Bakos HW, Henshaw RC, Mitchell M, Lane M. Paternal body mass index is associated with decreased blastocyst development and reduced live birth rates following assisted reproductive technology. *Fertil Steril*. 2011;95(5):1700-1704. doi:10.1016/j.fertnstert.2010.11.044.

102.    Palmer NO, Bakos HW, Fullston T, Lane M. Impact of obesity on male fertility, sperm function and molecular composition. *Spermatogenesis*. 2012;2(4):253-263. doi:10.4161/spmg.21362.

103.    Rittenberg V, Sobaleva S, Ahmad A, et al. Influence of BMI on risk of miscarriage after single blastocyst transfer. *Hum Reprod*. 2011;26(10):2642-2650. doi:10.1093/humrep/der254.

104.    Frisch RE. Body fat, menarche, fitness and fertility. *Hum Reprod*. 1987;2(6):521-533. http://www.ncbi.nlm.nih.gov/pubmed/3117838. Accessed July 14, 2017.

105.    Fertility Coalition. Fertility and a woman's weight. Your Fertility Website. https://yourfertility.org.au/for-women/weight-and-fertility/. Published 2018. Accessed August 7, 2018.

106.    Chavarro JE, Rich-Edwards JW, Rosner B, Willett WC. A prospective study of dairy foods intake and anovulatory infertility. *Hum Reprod*. 2007;22(5):1340-1347. doi:10.1093/humrep/dem019.

107.    Australian Government Department of Health. Make your move - sit less, be active for life! Physical Activity and Sedentary Behaviour Guidelines for Adults. http://www.health.gov.au/internet/main/publishing.nsf/content/health-pubhlth-strateg-phys-act-guidelines. Published 2014. Accessed July 17, 2017.

108.    Crespo NC, Mullane SL, Zeigler ZS, Buman MP, Gaesser GA. Effects of Standing and Light-Intensity Walking and Cycling on 24-h Glucose. *Med Sci Sports Exerc*. 2016;48(12):2503-2511. doi:10.1249/MSS.0000000000001062.

109.    Homer AR, Fenemor SP, Perry TL, et al. Regular activity breaks combined with physical activity improve postprandial plasma triglyceride, nonesterified fatty acid, and insulin responses in healthy, normal weight adults: A randomized crossover trial. *J Clin Lipidol*. June 2017. doi:10.1016/j.jacl.2017.06.007.

110.    Akhter S, Marcus M, Kerber RA, Kong M, Taylor KC. The impact of periconceptional maternal stress on fecundability. *Ann Epidemiol*. 2016;26(10):710-716. doi:10.1016/j.annepidem.2016.07.015.

111.    Kalantaridou SN, Makrigiannakis A, Zoumakis E, Chrousos GP. Stress and the female reproductive system. *J Reprod Immunol*. 2004;62(1-2):61-68. doi:10.1016/j.jri.2003.09.004.

112.    Bae J, Park S, Kwon JW. Factors associated with menstrual cycle irregularity and menopause. *BMC Womens Health*. 2018;18(1):1-11. doi:10.1186/s12905-018-0528-x.

113.    An Y, Sun Z, Li L, Zhang Y, Ji H. Relationship between psychological stress and reproductive outcome in women undergoing in vitro fertilization treatment: Psychological and neurohormonal assessment. *J Assist Reprod Genet*. 2013;30(1):35-41. doi:10.1007/s10815-012-9904-x.

114.    Prasad S, Tiwari M, Pandey AN, Shrivastav TG, Chaube SK. Impact of stress on oocyte quality and reproductive outcome. *J Biomed Sci*. 2016;23(1):19-23. doi:10.1186/s12929-016-0253-4.

115.    Ebbesen SMS, Zachariae R, Mehlsen MY, et al. Stressful life events are associated with a poor in-vitro fertilization (IVF) outcome: A prospective study. *Hum Reprod*. 2009;24(9):2173-2182. doi:10.1093/humrep/dep185.

116.    Fleming TP, Watkins AJ, Velazquez MA, et al. Origins of Lifetime Health Around the Time of Conception: Causes and Consequences. *Obstet Gynecol Surv*. 2018;73(10):555-557. doi:10.1097/OGX.0000000000000612.

117. McGonigal K. *The Upside of Stress: Why Stress Is Good for You, and How to Get Good at It*. New York, NY: Penguin Randomhouse LLC; 2015.

118. Domar AD, Clapp D, Slawsby EA, Dusek J, Kessel B, Freizinger M. Impact of group psychological interventions on pregnancy rates in infertile women. *Fertil Steril*. 2000;73(4):805-811. doi:S0015-0282(99)00493-8 [pii].

119. Clarke RN, Klock SC, Geoghegan A, Travassos DE. Relationship between psychological stress and semen quality among in-vitro fertilization patients. 1999;14(3):753-758.

120. Hilimire MR, DeVylder JE, Forestell CA. Fermented foods, neuroticism, and social anxiety: An interaction model. *Psychiatry Res*. 2015;228(2):203-208. doi:10.1016/j.psychres.2015.04.023.

121. Noori N, Bangash MY, Motaghinejad M, Hosseini P, Noudoost B. Kefir protective effects against nicotine cessation-induced anxiety and cognition impairments in rats. *Adv Biomed Res*. 2014;3:251. doi:10.4103/2277-9175.146377.

122. Trial DPC, Ostadrahimi A, Taghizadeh A, Mobasseri M. Effect of Probiotic Fermented Milk ( Kefir ) on Glycemic Control and Lipid Profile In Type 2 Diabetic Patients : A Randomized. 2015;44(2):228-237.

123. Cuddy A. *Your Body Language May Shape Who You Are*. Ted Talks; 2012. https://www.ted.com/talks/amy_cuddy_your_body_language_shapes_who_you_are.

124. Darbandi S, Darbandi M, Khorram Khorshid HR, Sadeghi MR. Yoga Can Improve Assisted Reproduction Technology Outcomes in Couples With Infertility. *Altern Ther Health Med*. November 2017. http://www.ncbi.nlm.nih.gov/pubmed/29112941. Accessed January 25, 2019.

125. Berk LS, Felten DL, Tan SA, Bittman BB, Westengard J. Modulation of neuroimmune parameters during the eustress of humor-associated mirthful laughter. *Altern Ther Health Med*. 2001;7(2):62-76.

126. Friedler S, Glasser S, Azani L, et al. The effect of medical clowning on pregnancy rates after in vitro fertilization and embryo transfer. *Fertil Steril*. 2011;95(6):2127-2130. doi:10.1016/j.fertnstert.2010.12.016.

127. Marlo H, Wagner MK. Expression of negative and positive events through writing: Implications for psychotherapy and health. *Psychol Health*. 1999;14(2):193-215. doi:10.1080/08870449908407323.

128. Baker FC, Driver HS. Circadian rhythms, sleep, and the menstrual cycle. *Sleep Med*. 2007;8(6):613-622. doi:10.1016/j.sleep.2006.09.011.

129. Taheri S, Lin L, Austin D, Young T, Mignot E. Short sleep duration is associated with reduced leptin, elevated ghrelin, and increased body mass index. *PLoS Med*. 2004;1(3):210-217. doi:10.1371/journal.pmed.0010062.

130. Dupuis L, Schuermann Y, Cohen T, et al. Role of leptin receptors in granulosa cells during ovulation. *Reproduction*. 2014;147(2):221-229. doi:10.1530/REP-13-0356.

131. Van Dongen HPA, Maislin G, Mullington JM, Dinges DF. The cumulative cost of additional wakefulness: dose-response effects on neurobehavioral functions and sleep physiology from chronic sleep restriction and total sleep deprivation. *Sleep*. 2003;26(2):117-126. doi:10.1001/archsurg.2011.121.

132. Leger D, Beck F, Richard JB, Sauvet F, Faraut B. The risks of sleeping "too much". Survey of a national representative sample of 24671 adults (INPES health barometer). *PLoS One*. 2014;9(9). doi:10.1371/journal.pone.0106950.

133. Barron ML. Light Exposure, Melatonin Secretion, and Menstrual Cycle Parameters: An Integrative Review. 2007:49-69.

134. Pilcher JJ, Michalowski KR, Carrigan RD. The prevalence of daytime napping and its relationship to nighttime sleep. *Behav Med*. 2001;27(2):71-76. doi:10.1080/08964280109595773.

135. Wong MY, Ree MJ, Lee CW. Enhancing CBT for Chronic Insomnia: A Randomised Clinical Trial of Additive Components of Mindfulness or Cognitive Therapy. *Clin Psychol Psychother*. 2016;23(5):377-385. doi:10.1002/cpp.1980.

136. Bijlsma N. *Healthy Home, Healthy Family*. Joshua Books; 2010.

137. American Chemical Society. CAS Content | The World's Largest Collection of Chemistry Insights. https://www.cas.org/about/cas-content. Accessed August 9, 2018.

138. Bergman Å, Heindel J, Jobling S, Kidd K, Zoeller RT. *State of the Science of Endocrine Disrupting Chemicals, 2012*. Vol 211.; 2012. doi:10.1016/j.toxlet.2012.03.020.

139. World Health Organization. *Identification of Risks from Exposure to ENDOCRINE-DISRUPTING CHEMICALS at the Country Level*.; 2014.

140. Diamanti-Kandarakis E, Bourguignon J-P, Giudice LC, et al. Endocrine-Disrupting Chemicals: An Endocrine Society Scientific Statement. *Endocr Rev*. 2009;30(4):293-342. doi:10.1210/er.2009-0002.

141. Ehrlich S, Williams PL, Missmer SA, et al. Urinary bisphenol A concentrations and early reproductive health outcomes among women undergoing IVF. *Hum Reprod*. 2012;27(12):3583-3592. doi:10.1093/humrep/des328.

142. Hart RJ, Doherty DA, Keelan JA, et al. The impact of antenatal Bisphenol A exposure on male reproductive function at 20–22 years of age. *Reprod Biomed Online*. 2018;36(3):340-347. doi:10.1016/j.rbmo.2017.11.009.

143. Ashiru O a, Odusanya OO. Fertility and occupational hazards: review of the literature. *Afr J Reprod Health.* 2009;13(1):159-165.

144. Thomas KW, Pellizzari ED, Perritt RL, Nelson WC. Effect of dry-cleaned clothes on tetrachloroethylene levels in indoor air, personal air, and breath for residents of several New Jersey homes. *J Expo Anal Environ Epidemiol.* 1991;1(4):475-490. http://www.ncbi.nlm.nih.gov/pubmed/1824329. Accessed August 27, 2017.

145. Ferguson KK, McElrath TF, Meeker JD. Environmental phthalate exposure and preterm birth. *JAMA Pediatr.* 2014;168(1):61-67. doi:10.1001/jamapediatrics.2013.3699.

146. Storyofstuffproject. *The Story of Cosmetics.* YouTube; 2010. https://www.youtube.com/watch?v=pfq000AF1i8.

147. Bijlsma N. Which Type of Water Filter. http://www.buildingbiology.com.au/hazards/which-type-of-water-filter.html. Published 2017. Accessed August 27, 2017.

148. Adams JA, Galloway TS, Mondal D, Esteves SC, Mathews F. Effect of mobile telephones on sperm quality: A systematic review and meta-analysis. Environ Int. 2014;70:106-112. doi:10.1016/j.envint.2014.04.015.

149. Avendano C, Mata A, Sanches Sarmiento CA, Doncel GF. Use of laptop computers connected to internet through Wi-Fi decreases human sperm motility and increases sperm DNA fragmentation. Fertil Steril. 2012;97(1):39-45. doi:10.1016/j.eururo.2012.09.017.

150. McIntosh T. Detoxification in Our Children. Brisbane; 2018.

151. Twigt JM, Bolhuis MEC, Steegers EAP, et al. The preconception diet is associated with the chance of ongoing pregnancy in women undergoing IVF/ICSI treatment. *Hum Reprod.* 2012;27(8):2526-2531. doi:10.1093/humrep/des157.

152. Vujkovic M, De Vries JH, Lindemans J, et al. The preconception Mediterranean dietary pattern in couples undergoing in vitro fertilization/intracytoplasmic sperm injection treatment increases the chance of pregnancy. *Fertil Steril.* 2010;94(6):2096-2101. doi:10.1016/j.fertnstert.2009.12.079.

153. Ricci E, Al-Beitawi S, Cipriani S, et al. Dietary habits and semen parameters: a systematic narrative review. *Andrology.* 2018;6(1):104-116. doi:10.1111/andr.12452.

154. Moran LJ, Myers J, Kenny LC, et al. Pre-pregnancy fast food and fruit intake is associated with time to pregnancy. *Hum Reprod.* 2018;33(6):1063-1070. doi:10.1093/humrep/dey079.

155.    Toledo E, Lopez-Del Burgo C, Ruiz-Zambrana A, et al. Dietary patterns and difficulty conceiving: A nested case-control study. *Fertil Steril*. 2011;96(5):1149-1153. doi:10.1016/j.fertnstert.2011.08.034.

156.    Braga DPAF, Halpern G, Setti AS, Figueira RCS, Iaconelli A, Borges E. The impact of food intake and social habits on embryo quality and the likelihood of blastocyst formation. *Reprod Biomed Online*. 2015;31(1):30-38. doi:10.1016/j.rbmo.2015.03.007.

157.    Chiu Y-H, Chavarro JE, Souter I. Diet and female fertility: doctor, what should I eat? *Fertil Steril*. 2018;110(4):560-569. doi:10.1016/j. fertnstert.2018.05.027.

158.    He F-J, Chen J-Q. Consumption of soybean, soy foods, soy isoflavones and breast cancer incidence: Differences between Chinese women and women in Western countries and possible mechanisms. *Food Sci Hum Wellness*. 2013;2(3-4):146-161. doi:10.1016/j.fshw.2013.08.002.

159.    Jefferson WN. Adult Ovarian Function Can Be Affected by High Levels of Soy. *J Nutr*. 2010;140(12):2322S-2325S. doi:10.3945/jn.110.123802.

160.    Zhang Z, Fulgoni VL, Kris-Etherton PM, Mitmesser SH. Dietary intakes of EPA and DHA omega-3 fatty acids among US childbearing-age and pregnant women: An analysis of NHANES 2001–2014. *Nutrients*. 2018;10(4). doi:10.3390/nu10040416.

161.    Coletta J, Bell S, Roman A. Omega-3 Fatty Acids and Pregnancy. *Rev Obs Gynecol*. 2010;3(4):163-171. doi:10.3909/riog0137.

162.    Attaman JA, Toth TL, Furtado J, Campos H, Hauser R, Chavarro JE. Dietary fat and semen quality among men attending a fertility clinic. *Hum Reprod*. 2012;27(5):1466-1474. doi:10.1093/humrep/des065.

163.    Hammiche F, Vujkovic M, Wijburg W, et al. Increased preconception omega-3 polyunsaturated fatty acid intake improves embryo morphology. *Fertil Steril*. 2011;95(5):1820-1823. doi:10.1016/j. fertnstert.2010.11.021.

164.    Robbins WA, Xun L, FitzGerald LZ, Esguerra S, Henning SM, Carpenter CL. Walnuts Improve Semen Quality in Men Consuming a Western-Style Diet: Randomized Control Dietary Intervention Trial1. *Biol Reprod*. 2012;87(4):1-8. doi:10.1095/biolreprod.112.101634.

165.    Wyatt KM, Harper DM. Review: Vitamin B6 is beneficial in the premenstrual syndrome. *Evid Based Med*. 1999;4(6):3-5.

166.    Fathizadeh N, Ebrahimi E, Valiani M, Tavakoli N, Hojat Yar M. Evaluating the effect of magnesium and magnesium plus vitamin B6 supplement on the severity of premenstrual syndrome. *Iran J Nurs Midwifery Res*. 2010;15(1):401-405.

167. Sampalis F, Bunea R, Pelland MF, Kowalski O, Duguet N, Dupuis S. Evaluation of the Effects of Neptune Krill Oil on the Management of Premenstrual Syndrome Krill Oil & PMS Evaluation of the Effects of Neptune Krill OilTM on the Management of Premenstrual Syndrome and Dysmenorrhea. *Altern Med Rev Altern Med Rev* ♦. 2003;8(2):171-179.

168. Pereira N. Revisiting the relationship between vitamin D and ovarian reserve. *Fertil Steril*. 2018;110(4):643. doi:10.1016/j.fertnstert.2018.07.001.

169. Teede HJ, Misso ML, Costello MF, et al. Recommendations from the international evidence-based guideline for the assessment and management of polycystic ovary syndrome. *Hum Reprod*. 2018;33(9):1602-1618. doi:10.1093/humrep/dey256.

170. Boyle J, Teede HJ. Polycystic ovary syndrome. *Aust Fam Physician*. 2012;41(10):752-756. http://www.nejm.org/doi/full/. Accessed March 12, 2014.

171. Jakubowicz D, Barnea M, Wainstein J, et al. Effects of caloric intake timing on insulin resistance and hyperandrogenism in lean women with polycystic ovary syndrome. *Clin Sci (Lond)*. 2013;125(9):423-432. doi:10.1042/CS20130071.

172. Norman RJ, Noakes M, Wu R, Davies MJ, Moran L, Wang JX. Improving reproductive performance in overweight/obese women with effective weight management. *Hum Reprod Update*. 2004;10(3):267-280. doi:10.1093/humupd/dmh018.

173. Sabatini L, Charles D, Thangaratinam S, et al. Overview of systematic reviews of non-pharmacological interventions in women with polycystic ovary syndrome. *Hum Reprod Update*. 2018;25(2):243-256. doi:10.1093/humupd/dmy045.

174. Birkenfeld A, Mukaida T, Minichiello L, Jackson M, Kase NG, Yemini M. Incidence of Autoimmune Antibodies in Failed Embryo Transfer Cycles. *Am J Reprod Immunol*. 1994;31(2-3):65-68. doi:10.1111/j.1600-0897.1994.tb00848.x.

175. Ohta A, Lukashev D, Jackson EK, Fredholm BB, Sitkovsky M. 1,3,7-Trimethylxanthine (Caffeine) May Exacerbate Acute Inflammatory Liver Injury By Weakening the Physiological Immunosuppressive Mechanism. *J Immunol*. 2007;179(11):7431-7438. doi:10.4049/jimmunol.179.11.7431.

176. Gold EB. The Timing of the Age at Which Natural Menopause Occurs. *Obstet Gynecol Clin North Am*. 2011;38(3):425-440. doi:10.1016/j.ogc.2011.05.002.

177.    The American College of Obstetricians and Gynecologists Committee on Gynecologic Practice. Committee Opinion: Female Age-Related Fertility Decline, Number 589.; 2014.

178.    UNSW School of Women's and Childrens Health. Module 3: Female Infertility, In: SWCH9004- Clinical Reproductive Medicine. 2013.

179.    The Fertility Society of Australia, Fertility Coalition. Age and reproductive outcomes. https://www.yourfertility.org.au/sites/default/files/2018-11/Age_and_reproductive_outcomes.pdf. Published 2018. Accessed February 2, 2019.

180.    Fertility Coalition. A man's age matters. Your Fertility Website. https://yourfertility.org.au/for-men/age/. Published 2017. Accessed September 19, 2017.

181.    FISCH H, HYUN G, GOLDEN R, HENSLE TW, OLSSON CA, LIBERSON GL. The Influence of Paternal Age on Down Syndrome. *J Urol.* 2003;169(6):2275-2278. doi:10.1097/01.ju.0000067958.36077.d8.

182.    Kleinhaus K, Perrin M, Friedlander Y, Paltiel O, Malaspina D, Harlap S. Paternal Age and Spontaneous Abortion. *Obstet Gynecol.* 2006;108(2):369-377. doi:10.1097/01.AOG.0000224606.26514.3a.

183.    Malaspina D, Harlap S, Fennig S, et al. Advancing paternal age and the risk of schizophrenia. *Arch Gen Psychiatry.* 2001;58(4):361-367. http://www.ncbi.nlm.nih.gov/pubmed/11296097. Accessed September 19, 2017.

184.    Fitzgerald O, Paul R, Harris K, Chambers G. *Assisted Reproductive Technology in Australia and New Zealand*; 2016. https://npesu.unsw.edu.au/sites/default/files/npesu/surveillances/Assisted%20Reproductive%20Technology%20in%20Australia%20and%20New%20Zealand%202016.pdf.

185.    Massaro PA, Maclellan DL, Anderson PA, Romao RLP. Does intracytoplasmic sperm injection pose an increased risk of genitourinary congenital malformations in offspring compared to in vitro fertilization? A systematic review and meta-analysis. *J Urol.* 2015;193(5):1837-1842. doi:10.1016/j.juro.2014.10.113.

186.    Rowley MJ, Teshima F, Heller CG. Duration of Transit of Spermatozoa through the Human Male Ductular System. *Fertil Steril.* 1970;21(5):390-396. doi:10.1016/S0015-0282(16)37502-1.

187.    Howe G, Westhoff C, Vessey M, Yeates D. Effects of age, cigarette smoking, and other factors on fertility: findings in a large prospective study. *Br Med J (Clin Res Ed).* 1985;290(6483):1697-1700. doi:10.1136/bmj.290.6483.1697.

188. Kalmbach KH, Antunes D, Wang F, Buldo-Licciardi J, Kramer Y, Keefe D. Oocyte telomere length is associated with ovarian reserve and ovarian response in female infertility patients. *Fertil Steril.* 2013;100(3):S45. doi:10.1016/j.fertnstert.2013.07.1817.

189. Liu S, CJ Z, HY P, et al. Association study of telomere length with idiopathic male infertility. *HEREDITAS(Beijing).* 2015;37(11):1137-1142. http://www.chinagene.cn/EN/abstract/abstract21537.shtml.

190. Albizua I, Rambo-Martin R, Allen E, He W, Amin A, Sherman S. Association between telomere length and chromosome 21 nondisjunction in the oocyte. *Hum Genet.* 2015;134(0):1263-1270. doi:10.1111/obr.12065.Variation.

191. Hanna CW, Bretherick KL, Gair JL, Fluker MR, Stephenson MD, Robinson WP. Telomere length and reproductive aging. *Hum Reprod.* 2009;24(5):1206-1211. doi:10.1093/humrep/dep007.

192. Biron-Shental T, Sukenik-Halevy R, Sharon Y, et al. Short telomeres may play a role in placental dysfunction in preeclampsia and intrauterine growth restriction. *Am J Obstet Gynecol.* 2010;202(4):381.e1-381.e7. doi:10.1016/j.ajog.2010.01.036.

193. Biron-Shental T, Sukenik Halevy R, Goldberg-Bittman L, Kidron D, Fejgin MD, Amiel A. Telomeres are shorter in placental trophoblasts of pregnancies complicated with intrauterine growth restriction (IUGR). *Early Hum Dev.* 2010;86(7):451-456. doi:10.1016/j.earlhumdev.2010.06.002.

194. Hallows SE, Regnault TRH, Betts DH. Hepatocyte telomere shortening and senescence are general markers of human liver cirrhosis. *J Pregnancy.* 2012;2012. doi:10.1155/2012/638476.

195. Wentzensen IM, Mirabello L, Pfeiffer RM, Savage SA. The association of telomere length and cancer: A meta-analysis. *Cancer Epidemiol Biomarkers Prev.* 2011;20(6):1238-1250. doi:10.1158/1055-9965.EPI-11-0005.

196. Bakaysa SL, Mucci LA, Slagboom PE, et al. Telomere length predicts survival independent of genetic influences. *Aging Cell.* 2007;6(6):769-774. doi:10.1111/j.1474-9726.2007.00340.x.

197. Ornish D, Lin J, Chan JM, et al. Effect of comprehensive lifestyle changes on telomerase activity and telomere length in men with biopsy-proven low-risk prostate cancer: 5-year follow-up of a descriptive pilot study. *Lancet Oncol.* 2013;14(11):1112-1120. doi:10.1016/S1470-2045(13)70366-8.

198. Tolahunase MR, Sagar R, Chaurasia P, Dada R. Impact of yoga- and meditation-based lifestyle intervention on depression, quality of life, and cellular aging in infertile couples. *Fertil Steril.* 2018;110(4):e67. doi:10.1016/j.fertnstert.2018.07.203.

199. Safdar A, Little JP, Stokl AJ, Hettinga BP, Akhtar M, Tarnopolsky MA. Exercise increases mitochondrial PGC-1α content and promotes nuclear-mitochondrial cross-talk to coordinate mitochondrial biogenesis. *J Biol Chem*. 2011;286(12):10605-10617. doi:10.1074/jbc.M110.211466.

200. Nassan FL, Chavarro JE, Tanrikut C. Diet and men's fertility: does diet affect sperm quality? *Fertil Steril*. 2018;110(4):570-577. doi:10.1016/j.fertnstert.2018.05.025.

201. Yang Y, Luo Y, Yuan J, et al. Association between maternal, fetal and paternal MTHFR gene C677T and A1298C polymorphisms and risk of recurrent pregnancy loss: a comprehensive evaluation. *Arch Gynecol Obstet*. 2016;293(6):1197-1211. doi:10.1007/s00404-015-3944-2.

202. Zhu X, Liu Z, Zhang M, Gong R, Xu Y, Wang B. Association of the methylenetetrahydrofolate reductase gene *C677T* polymorphism with the risk of male infertility: a meta-analysis. *Ren Fail*. 2016;38(2):185-193. doi:10.3109/0886022X.2015.1111086.

203. Ling X, Zhang G, Chen Q, et al. Shorter sperm telomere length in association with exposure to polycyclic aromatic hydrocarbons: Results from the MARHCS cohort study in Chongqing, China and in vivo animal experiments. *Environ Int*. 2016;95:79-85. doi:10.1016/j.envint.2016.08.001.

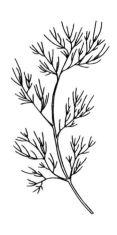

Yay for us!! We did it!
6+ years in the making,
we hope it has been
worth it for you!

Please do be in touch
to let us know how
you are going with
it and if we can help.

———————————————

Best wishes from all of us at
Fertile Ground Health Group